The Scientific Basis of Joint Replacement

Edited by

S. A. V. Swanson, DSc (Eng), PhD, DIC, ACGI, MIMechE
Professor of Biomechanics at Imperial College in the University of London
Director, Biomechanics Unit, Imperial College, London

and

M. A. R. Freeman, MD, MB, BCh, BA, FRCS
Consultant Orthopaedic Surgeon, The London Hospital
Director, Bone and Joint Research Unit, The London Hospital Medical College
Director, Biomechanics Unit, Imperial College, London

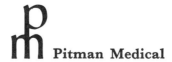
Pitman Medical

First published 1977

PITMAN MEDICAL PUBLISHING CO LTD
42 Camden Road, Tunbridge Wells,
Kent TN1 2QD

Associated Companies

UNITED KINGDOM
Pitman Publishing Ltd, London
Focal Press Ltd, London

USA
Pitman Publishing Corporation, California
Fearon Publishers Inc, California

AUSTRALIA
Pitman Publishing Pty Ltd, Melbourne

CANADA
Pitman Publishing, Toronto
Copp Clark Publishing, Toronto

EAST AFRICA
Sir Isaac Pitman and Sons Ltd, Nairobi

SOUTH AFRICA
Pitman Publishing Co SA (Pty) Ltd, Johannesburg

NEW ZEALAND
Pitman Publishing NZ Ltd, Wellington

© Pitman Medical Publishing Co Ltd 1977

ISBN: 0 272 79380 9
Cat. No. 21 1002 81

Set in 10/11 point Intertype Baskerville at
Western Printing Services, Bristol, and printed by
photolithography and bound in Great Britain at
The Pitman Press, Bath, Avon.

Contents

Acknowledgement

The authors are grateful for permission to reproduce in this book some of their illustrations which they have published elsewhere.

Figures 2.11–2.13: B. Weightman (1976) The stresses in total hip prosthesis femoral stems: a comparative study. In, *Engineering in Medicine*, Vol. 2. Berlin, Springer-Verlag.

Figures 3.9 & 3.10: B. Weightman et al. (1972) Lubrication mechanisms of hip joint replacement prostheses. *Journal of Lubrication Technology (Trans. ASME)* 94, 131.

Figure 3.12: B. Weightman et al. (1973) A comparative study of total hip replacement prostheses. *Journal of Biomechanics* 6, 299.

Figures 4.1.–4.31: B. Vernon-Roberts and M. A. R. Freeman (1976) Morphological and analytical studies of the tissues adjacent to joint prostheses: investigations into the causes of loosening of prostheses. In, *Engineering in Medicine*, Vol. 2. Berlin, Springer-Verlag.

A Surgeon's Introduction

This book is concerned with the sciences basic to total joint replacement. Thus it has been written by engineers and a pathologist. Since the application of the basic knowledge is a matter for orthopaedic surgeons, it is essential that the relevance of the subjects dealt with and the subjects themselves should be clear to clinicians. To ensure this, each chapter has been closely edited and in parts written by an orthopaedic surgeon with a special interest in this topic. Since each chapter has been drafted alternately by a basic scientist and a clinician, the chapters as they now stand can be viewed as representing the end point of a clinical and scientific dialogue.

To write a book by this technique is only possible if all the authors and editors have close day-to-day contact with each other and are actively engaged in the problems of prosthetic design, testing, manufacture and implantation. In the case of this book these conditions are met since three of us (Professor S. A. V. Swanson, M. A. R. Freeman and Dr B. Weightman) direct and are on the staff of the Biomechanics Unit at Imperial College, whilst at the time of writing two of us (M. A. R. Freeman and Dr B. Vernon-Roberts) directed the Bone and Joint Research Unit at The London Hospital, both institutions heavily engaged in the joint replacement field.

This book is concerned with basic principles, not with the details of prosthetic design. Thus the reader will not find here, for example, a detailed critique of each and every prosthesis for the replacement of the hip, but will find sufficient information to enable him to judge for himself which prostheses are good, which bad and which have indistinguishable merits.

Prostheses are artefacts and therefore the first consideration must be with the properties of the materials of which they are made. This topic is dealt with in Chapter 1 whilst in Chapter 2 the mechanical interaction of these materials with their environment is considered. Since in the technique of total joint replacement two or more bearing surfaces are replaced, the materials react not only with their environment but also with each other in ways governed by considerations of lubrication and wear, topics covered in Chapter 3.

The interactions between the tissues and an implant are considered from the biological point of view in Chapter 4 and then from the mechanical point of view in Chapter 5. Finally, the last two chapters (Chapters 6 and 7) deal with the practical aspects of manufacturing implants and controlling their quality.

This field is changing rapidly and therefore it must be accepted that this book will date. Nevertheless, the Editors feel that there is now sufficient firm ground to make this book valuable in the long-term. Certainly the enormous clinical importance of joint replacement makes it urgent that it be placed upon a secure scientific footing. We hope that this volume is a step in that direction.

Properties of Materials

PROSTHESES for the replacement of joints must be able to withstand the loads applied to them in the body. In other words, the stresses produced in an artificial joint must neither fracture the prosthesis nor deform it excessively. The design of any joint component therefore involves a knowledge of the properties of different materials and an analysis of the stresses which will be produced in the implant. These two interrelated topics are dealt with in this chapter and the next; the present chapter is concerned with the basic material properties relevant to total joint replacements, while the problem of analysing the stresses produced by different types of applied load is discussed in the following chapter.

1 BASIC MATERIAL PROPERTIES

1.1 Tensile Properties

The tensile test is perhaps the most widely used test of the mechanical properties of materials. In this test, a specimen of the material is stretched, usually at a constant rate, and both the tensile force being applied and the elongation produced are measured. Graphs of load (force) against elongation may be plotted, but it is more usual to convert these quantities to stress and strain respectively so that the graphs are independent of specimen size. Stress is defined as the ratio of load to cross-sectional area (it is common practice to use the original cross-sectional area of the specimen rather than the reduced cross-section produced by elongation and to call the resulting stress the 'engineering stress'), and 'engineering strain' is defined as the ratio of the change in length to the original length.

Although different types of material behave differently in the tensile test, the various characteristic behaviours can be discussed with reference to the stress–strain curve shown in Fig. 1.1. During the first part of the test (O–A, Fig. 1.1) most materials behave elastically. That is, if the test is stopped and the load released, the specimen returns to its original dimensions. With most metals and ceramics the relationship between stress and strain in this elastic region is linear and the slope of the curve is known as Young's modulus, E, of the material.

Figure 1.1.
Schematic stress–strain curve.

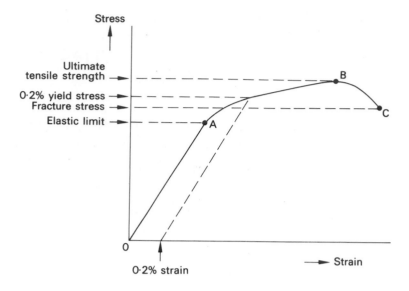

The application of tensile stress to the specimen affects the material in two ways. Firstly, it tends to pull the atoms of the material apart on planes perpendicular to the direction of loading. Secondly, because the applied tensile stress produces shear stresses in the material which have a maximum value on planes at 45° to the direction of loading (see Chapter 2, section 1.1), there is a tendency for atoms to slip over each other along these planes and take up new positions. Therefore, as the applied load is increased during the tensile test, a stress level is eventually reached (point A, Fig. 1.1) at which either fracture or shear slip occurs.

If the magnitude of the induced shear stress reaches the level required to produce slipping before the tensile stress reaches the cohesive strength of the material, large non-reversible or *plastic* deformations occur as the applied load increases further. That is, the material exceeds its *elastic limit* and the specimen does not return to its original dimensions if the load is released. If the material 'strain hardens' (or 'work hardens') further elongation requires an increasing stress and the slope of the stress–strain curve in this region (A–B, Fig. 1.1) provides a measure of the material's strain hardenability. Eventually the engineering stress reaches a maximum value known as the *ultimate tensile strength* of the material (point B, Fig. 1.1). Some materials then develop a neck at which the cross-sectional area of the specimen is reduced locally. When this occurs the engineering stress falls with further elongation until the specimen fractures (point C, Fig. 1.1). In these materials, the *fracture stress* is less than the ultimate tensile strength. Materials which exhibit plastic behaviour are known as *ductile* materials, and the percentage strain or elongation of a specimen at fracture (usually measured by fitting the broken parts together after fracture) is a measure of ductility.

Materials which do not deform plastically before fracture, because the applied tensile stress reaches the cohesive strength of the material before slipping can occur, are classified as *brittle*. For such a material, the tensile stress–strain curve ends at point A in Fig. 1.1.

All materials contain defects which produce localised stresses of much greater magnitude than the average stress applied to the specimen. Brittle materials are generally weak in tension because fracture occurs in these regions of higher than average stress and rapidly propagates across the whole specimen. The same materials can, however, be much stronger in compression, for the simple reason that compressive stresses do not pull the atoms apart. In ductile materials high tensile stresses around defects produce localised plastic deformation. Since this effectively prevents crack propagation, ductile materials are not seriously weaker in tension than in compression.

Of the three measures of a material's tensile strength so far discussed (namely, elastic limit, ultimate tensile strength, and fracture strength), the elastic limit is the most important because most engineering structures are designed to remain within the elastic range. Because it is often difficult in practice to establish accurately the transition from elastic to plastic behaviour, it is common practice to specify a material's 0·2 per cent yield stress. This, sometimes called the 0·2 per cent proof stress or the 0·2 per cent offset yield stress, is the stress corresponding to a plastic (non-recoverable) strain of 0·2 per cent (as indicated in Fig. 1.1), and is close enough to the elastic limit to be used as a basis for design.

The above discussion covers the behaviour of metals, ranging from ductile copper to brittle cast iron, and brittle ceramics, but polymeric materials must be given special mention. Polymers behave partly like viscous liquids and partly like elastic solids. This so-called *viscoelastic* behaviour means that the deformation of polymers under load is a function of time as well as of stress. When a constant load is applied to a polymer specimen there is an initial deformation, as in an elastic material, followed by a deformation which gradually increases with time (*creep*). In tensile tests the viscoelastic nature of polymers is reflected in the variation of the measured properties with strain rate. In general, as the rate of elongation increases, the tensile strength and stiffness (Young's modulus) increase while the total elongation at break (ductility) decreases. Many metals also exhibit time-dependent behaviour, but at the temperatures relevant to the use of implants the effects are negligible.

1.2 Fracture

In the same way that materials can be described as either ductile or brittle, fracture (i.e. the separation of a body into two or more parts) can be classified as either ductile or brittle. Ductile fracture is preceded by large plastic deformations. The fracture of ductile metals is characterised by slow crack propagation and the fracture surface is generally dull and fibrous in appearance. Brittle fracture of metals occurs rapidly, without any appreciable plastic deformation, along certain crystal planes called *cleavage planes*, and this gives a granular appearance to the fracture surface.

Materials which are normally ductile can under certain conditions exhibit brittle fracture. When a material is subjected to tensile stresses in three mutually perpendicular directions, instead of in one direction as in the tensile test, the magnitude of the internally produced shear stresses is reduced. If the shear stresses are reduced sufficiently, the cohesive strength of the material will be exceeded before the plastic yield (shear) strength, and brittle fracture will occur without plastic deformation. A state of triaxial tension occurs, for example, at the tip of a notch or crack in a specimen loaded in simple tension. Decreasing temperature and increasing strain rate can also produce a transition from ductile to brittle behaviour, so that the combination of a notch and high strain rate, for example, can produce a brittle fracture in a normally ductile material.

1.3 The Hardness Test

The hardness of a material largely determines its machinability and its resistance to scratching, wear and penetration. The standard methods of measuring hardness, including the Brinell, Vickers and Rockwell tests, involve pressing a hard indenter into a flat surface of the material and measuring a particular dimension of the resulting impression. The ratio of load to cross-sectional area (calculated from the measured dimension) gives an empirical hardness number which has the dimensions of stress.

Since hardness tests generally produce plastic deformation, there is often a good correlation between hardness values and the properties determined in a tensile test. The speed with which hardness tests can be conducted and their non-destructive nature explain why they are frequently used for routine examinations such as the quality control of finished products.

The indentation hardness test is also of great importance in the study of the friction and wear characteristics of materials (see Chapter 3). When pressed together, solid bodies make contact at asperities on their surfaces and the similarity between this situation and hardness testing means that hardness is perhaps the most relevant mechanical property when two materials are in sliding contact.

1.4 Fatigue

Fatigue is an engineering term used to describe the failure of a material produced by a fluctuating stress. The stress required to produce fatigue failure, if applied a sufficient number of times, is often much lower than that required to fracture the material on a single application.

Most machine elements are subjected to fluctuating loads and over 80 per cent of all operating failures in general engineering are caused by fatigue. Although the stress cycles in these real situations are usually extremely complex, basic information about a material's fatigue properties can be obtained in the laboratory with simplified tests.

Figure 1.2 shows the machine for one such test. Round-sectioned, waisted specimens are rotated at high speed in a chuck attached to the shaft of an electric motor. A weight is hung at the other end of the specimen by means of a ball-bearing load carrier so that during each revolution all points on the circumference of the specimen are subjected to a stress varying sinusoidally from tension to compression. By testing a large number of specimens at different loads a fatigue graph of stress versus number of cycles to failure (S–N or S–$\log N$) is produced. Typical fatigue plots are shown in Fig. 1.3.

Certain materials (for example, some steels and titanium alloys) will not break if the magnitude of the fluctuating stress is below a certain value, called the *fatigue limit*, however many cycles of stress are applied; these materials have an 'infinite' fatigue life. Most materials, however, do not exhibit this phenomenon and may fail eventually even at low stress. In most practical cases a fatigue life of 100 million (10^8) cycles is more than sufficient and it is common practice to specify a material's fatigue strength (or endurance limit) as the stress which will produce fracture only after this number of cycles.

Figure 1.2.
One type of fatigue testing machine (rotating bending).

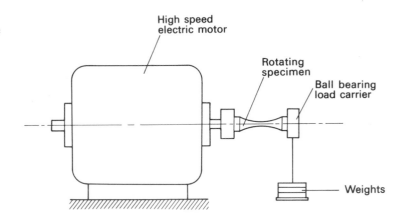

Figure 1.3.
Typical fatigue curves.

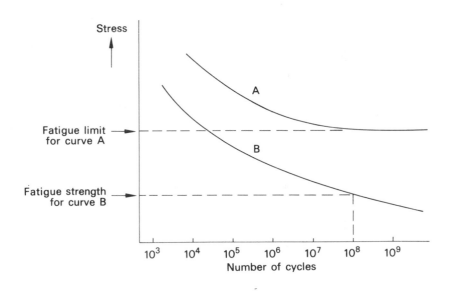

Many factors affect the results of laboratory fatigue tests and considerable scatter is normally found. Fatigue cracks usually start at the surface of a specimen, particularly when the stress is a maximum at the surface as in the rotating bending test, and for this reason surface finish has a very marked effect on fatigue results; the better the surface finish the longer the fatigue life. The test environment is important since corrosion can both initiate fatigue cracks (by producing pits in the surface) and accelerate their propagation (by attacking at the crack tip). Even in mildly corrosive environments the fatigue life of most metals and alloys is reduced, and alloys which exhibit a fatigue limit in dry air cease to do so. (See sections 1.5 and 1.6, below.)

The simple stress cycle applied to specimens in the rotating bending type of laboratory test (i.e. sinusoidal about a zero mean stress) does not represent most practical situations. Other tests in which a static load is superimposed on the fluctuating stress, so that the mean is no longer zero, have shown that an applied static tensile load decreases fatigue life and an applied static compressive load extends fatigue life. One reason for this is that a tensile stress tends to open surface cracks whereas a compressive stress tends to close them.

In practical situations fatigue fracture is usually initiated at localised regions of high stress caused by sudden changes in geometry. Stress concentrations are produced by such obvious changes in geometry as keyways, hole, notches and screw threads, but tool marks, scratches, sharp edges and engraved letters can also act as stress raisers.

On a macroscopic scale the fatigue-fractured surface of a metallic component normally consists of two distinct regions (indicated in Fig. 1.4): (1) a relatively smooth area with concentric markings, variously called conchoidal, clam-shell, oyster-shell, beach, or ripple marks; and (2) a region of either granular or fibrous appearance. The relatively smooth region is produced by the slow propagation of the fatigue crack and the clam-shell marks indicate the various positions at which the crack has stopped as it propagates intermittently through the component in response to the varying applied load. It is often possible to locate the origin (or origins) of the fracture from the clam-shell markings. Eventually, the remaining cross-sectional area can no longer support the applied load and rapid fracture occurs. This produces an area granular in appearance if the final fracture occurs in a brittle manner, or fibrous in appearance if ductile fracture occurs. In the latter case this region may also show evidence of large-scale plastic deformation. With some materials a very small fatigue crack may be sufficient to produce brittle fracture and the whole fracture surface may have the granular appearance characteristic of brittle fracture.

Fatigue fracture is not completely understood, but is generally taken to be initiated by a shear mechanism which produces microslip bands on the component surface. Eventually microcracks develop and these coalesce into a fatigue crack. The initial formation of this crack can take up to 90 per cent of the total fatigue life of the component and produces a small lip (shear lip) at the initiation site. After initiation the crack propagates relatively slowly by a process of plastic deformation, leaving concentric fatigue striations as it advances during each cyclic application of load. As the crack progresses the stress on the remaining cross-section increases and the resulting increase in crack propagation rate is shown by the increased spacing of the fatigue striations. On a microscopic scale, then, the observable characteristics of fatigue fracture are microslip lines on the component surface, a shear lip at the initiation site, and fatigue striations on the fracture surface.

Figure 1.4.
Schematic diagram of a fatigue-fracture surface.

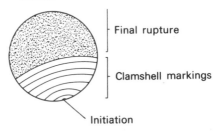

Final rupture

Clamshell markings

Initiation

1.5 Corrosion

Metals corrode in aqueous environments by an electrochemical mechanism. When a pure metal is immersed in a solution there is a tendency for metal atoms in the surface of the electrode to go into solution as positively charged ions. This reaction produces an excess of negatively charged electrons on the electrode which opposes further dissolution. Eventually an equilibrium is reached when the electrode potential of the metal is sufficient to counteract its further dissolution.

Different metals have different tendencies to dissolve and therefore reach different equilibrium potentials. When two such metals are in contact in solution (Fig. 1.5a), electrons flow from the metal with the more negative potential (i.e. more electrons) to the other. The first metal no longer has sufficient electrons to counteract metallic dissolution and the reaction proceeds. This metal has become an anode. The other metal now has an excess of electrons which are used in a reduction reaction. This is often the reduction of dissolved oxygen from the solution or the liberation of hydrogen gas. The second metal has become a cathode. The process is galvanic corrosion and it is always liable to occur when dissimilar metals are in contact. Essentially the same mechanism can occur with metals containing impurities or inclusions, with alloys having their constituents non-uniformly distributed, or with soldered and welded joints, since any differences of composition can lead to one area becoming anodic with respect to another.

Galvanic corrosion is particularly dangerous when the area of the anodic site is small compared with the area of the cathode. This is because the corrosion attack is concentrated and consequently the mechanical strength of a component can be significantly reduced by only a small loss of material.

Anodic and cathodic areas are produced on metals by other mechanisms. As a general rule, oxygen is required for the continuation of corrosion in neutral salt solutions but the supply of oxygen may vary over the surface of a component. Such variations in oxygen concentration can lead to corrosion, since regions with low concentrations become anodic with respect to regions of higher concentrations (Fig. 1.5b). Crevice corrosion (Fig. 1.5c), which is initiated by the exhaustion of oxygen within a narrow crevice, is a common and particularly dangerous example of this mechanism since the active corrosion is concentrated on a small area within the crevice.

Certain metals and alloys, including those used in orthopaedic surgery, are highly corrosion resistant because of an inert film of metal compound (usually an oxide) which forms on the surface. The inert layer is termed the *passivation* layer and such metals are known as *passive metals*. Unfortunately, however, passivity can break down in certain conditions. The passivating film itself may be susceptible to some forms of chemical attack, and chloride ions are particularly dangerous in this respect. The film may be damaged mechanically, by scratching for example, and if it cannot repair itself, active corrosion will occur at the exposed metal surface (Fig. 1.5d). Passive metals are susceptible to crevice corrosion since the lack of oxygen at the base of a crevice can eventually make the material here an anode. In chloride-containing solutions the resulting corrosion reaction can produce hydrochloric acid, and this accelerates the corrosion process. Crevice corrosion can also be initiated by slight relative movement between two components forming a crevice; for example, a screw head in a countersunk hole. The fretting motion mechanically damages the passivation layer and, if the long narrow electrolytic path of the crevice restricts oxygen diffusion so that repassivation cannot take place, active corrosion ensues.

Corrosion is an electrochemical process and can, therefore, occur only in metallic materials. However, both polymers and ceramics can react chemically with their environments with a subsequent reduction in mechanical properties, and this degradation can be thought of as being analogous to metallic corrosion.

Polymers can be degraded by heat, by radiation, by oxygen and oxidising agents, and by water. Although the mechanisms differ, the degradation process usually involves changes in molecular structure such as the shortening of molecular chains or a change in the degree of cross-linking between chains.

Little is known about the degradation of ceramics. Although as a class of materials they are noted for their chemical inertness, some ceramics will react with their environment (by oxidation and hydration, for example) and a careful choice of material is required for any particular application.

1.6 Corrosion-fatigue

Corrosion-fatigue occurs when a metal is subjected to a fluctuating stress in a corrosive environment. Pits or crevices produced by corrosion act as stress raisers and accelerate fatigue crack initiation. While it is obvious that this mechanism will reduce the fatigue life of a component, experiments have shown that the combined effect of corrosion and fatigue is greater than the effect of corrosion followed by fatigue. One reason for this is that the initial shear slipping at the surface which occurs in fatigue exposes bare metal (i.e. metal without a passivation layer) to the corrosive environment and hence accelerates the corrosion attack (Fig. 1.5e). A second reason is that the corrosion which occurs within the fatigue crack as it propagates increases the rate of propagation.

Metals which have a fatigue limit in air (Fig. 1.3, curve A) will fracture at stresses below this level in a corrosive environment, and fatigue curves obtained from tests in a corrosive environment usually do not show a fatigue limit; i.e. like curve B in Fig. 1.3.

In any examination of a failed component the presence of corrosion pits near the fracture initiation site is a strong indication that corrosion-fatigue was the mechanism of fracture. However, such pits may not be visible under a light microscope and the amount of material removed by corrosion may be so small that the component shows no obvious sign of corrosion.

Just as polymers and ceramics are degraded in certain environments by a process analogous to metallic corrosion, their fatigue strengths can be reduced in the presence of degrading environments in a manner analogous to corrosion-fatigue. The phenomenon has been variously termed environmental fatigue, degradative fatigue and stress-enhanced reactivity, and in polymers appears to be the result of an increased susceptibility to degradation produced by the stretching of molecular bonds.

Figure 1.5.
Corrosion and corrosion-fatigue.

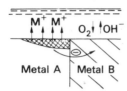

(a) Galvanic corrosion

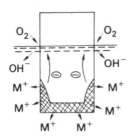

(b) Differential oxygenation

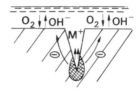

(c) Crevice corrosion

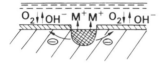

(d) Local breakdown of passive film (without repair)

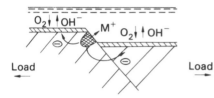

(e) Corrosion fatigue

2 MATERIALS USED IN TOTAL JOINT REPLACEMENTS

2.1 General Considerations

Table 1.1 lists some of the mechanical properties of materials which are used, or have been used, in total joint replacements. For comparison and reference polymethylmethacrylate bone cement and cortical bone are included.

Since metals, polymers and ceramics have widely different mechanical, chemical and electrochemical properties, it is perhaps surprising to see that all three classes of material are used. Before discussing each particular material in detail, therefore, it is important to realise why each type is used and what limitations their properties impose on their use.

Total joint replacements must be able to withstand the loads applied to them in the body; they must be resistant to corrosion and corrosion-fatigue; and they must have bearing surfaces giving low friction and wear. Furthermore, any corrosion products and wear debris must be well tolerated by the body. At the present time no one material can satisfy all of these requirements and for this reason different materials and different combinations of materials are used in attempts to produce the best possible total joint replacements.

Metallic materials are used because they, and only they, have the tensile, compressive and fatigue strengths required for such highly stressed parts as the femoral stems of hip prostheses. Few pure metals have the necessary combination of properties, but alloys of two or more metals often have better properties and are widely used in general engineering as well as for making implants. Thus stainless steel (essentially iron with the addition of carbon, chromium and nickel) has good mechanical properties and considerable resistance to corrosion. Titanium is unusual in having a useful combination of mechanical properties and corrosion resistance; but titanium alloyed

9

with, for example, aluminium and vanadium is better. Unfortunately, metals and alloys have a number of disadvantages. Firstly, they are liable to corrode, and this problem restricts the number of suitable metals to those listed in Table 1.1. Secondly, of the metals and alloys listed in Table 1.1 only cast cobalt–chromium alloy on itself is capable of providing a usable bearing for total joint replacements; all of the other metal-on-metal combinations produce prohibitively high friction and wear.

Polymers are used in total joint replacements because even the frictional forces in all-cobalt–chromium alloy prostheses are thought to contribute to loosening in some cases and because the wear products from such prostheses may have unacceptable biological properties; metal-on-polymer bearings produce lower friction (see Chapter 3, section 2.2) and their wear products appear to be less active biologically (see Chapter 4). Although most total joint replacements now contain a polymer component it is important to realise that the mechanical properties of polymers prevent their being used in highly stressed situations. Not only are their yield stresses low, but their viscoelastic (time-dependent) behaviour under load means that the stresses on them must be kept below the yield stress values in order to avoid creep.

The increasing interest in the use of ceramics is based on a number of factors. For example, certain ceramics appear to offer a combination of chemical inertness, low wear rates, low friction, and innocuous wear debris. While these properties make ceramics potentially attractive materials for the bearing surfaces of total joint replacements, their wider use is restricted by their extremely brittle behaviour which means that they cannot be used where significant tensile stresses are likely to be encountered.

In summary, metals and metallic alloys are used for the highly stressed parts of total joint replacements especially those which are stressed in tension, certain polymeric materials are now widely used to provide low-friction bearing surfaces, and certain ceramics appear to offer the possibility of a low volume of chemically inert wear debris. Since friction and wear are discussed in Chapter 3 and tissue tolerance in Chapter 4, the remaining sections of this chapter concentrate on the static strength, the fatigue strength, and the corrosion and corrosion-fatigue resistance of the metallic materials listed in Table 1.1. Comments on the properties of polymers and ceramics are made where appropriate.

2.2 Static Mechanical Properties

Most total joint replacement metallic components in present use are made of annealed stainless steel, cast cobalt–chromium alloy, or titanium. The other metallic alloys listed in Table 1.1 are either less commonly used in total joint replacements or are used for other types of surgical implant.

Annealed stainless steel, cast cobalt–chromium alloy and titanium have similar ultimate tensile strengths. However, yield stress is more important than ultimate tensile strength, and annealed stainless steel will yield (permanently deform) at a significantly lower stress than the other two materials. This means that an annealed stainless steel component requires a larger cross-sectional area than a similar cobalt–chromium alloy or titanium component if it is to avoid its inherently greater risk of plastic deformation.

Titanium and its alloys have moduli of elasticity approximately half those of the other alloys (100 GN/m² compared with approximately 200 GN/m²). As is shown in Chapter 2, section 3.2, the proportion of the load across a joint replacement transmitted through its intramedullary stem (where one exists) depends on the relative stiffnesses of the stem and the bone, and the stiffness of the stem is partly determined by the modulus of its material. It follows that titanium and the titanium alloys are slightly better for joint replacement stems than the other metals since their moduli are nearer to that of cortical bone (about 20 GN/m²). This consideration applies to load-sharing in general, not only to intramedullary stems.

Table 1.1   Selected Mechanical Properties of Materials Used in Total Joint Replacements

Material	Type and condition	Ultimate tensile strength MN/m²	Tensile yield stress MN/m²	Young's modulus GN/m²	Elongation at fracture %	Com-pressive strength MN/m²	Vickers hardness MN/m²	Fatigue strength (10^8 cycles) MN/m²
Stainless steel	316, 316L. Annealed	520–620	250–330	200	75–36		1400–1800	245–300
Cobalt–chromium alloy	Cast	650–750	440–570	200	8		3000–4000	235–275
Titanium, pure	Annealed	550–620	480–510	100	15–20		2400	250–280
Stainless steel	316, 316L. Cold worked	1000–1500	770–1370	200	8		3200	300
Cobalt–chromium alloy	'Wrought'. Cold worked	1000–1700	500–1300	230	9		4500	480
Cobalt–nickel alloy	MP 35 N Hot-forged	850–1200	650–1000	230	35–55		3000–4000	540–600
Titanium alloy	6 Al, 4V. Annealed	930	825	100	10–15		3500	400–440
Aluminium oxide ceramic	Al$_2$O$_3$	270	—	350	0	4000	20000	NA
Polyethylene	High molecular weight, RCH 1000	43	22	0·5	450	20		NA
Polyamide	Nylon 66	85	NA	3	40–80	NA		NA
Polyacetal	Delrin	70	NA	3	75	NA		NA
Polyester	Polyethylene terephthalate	80	NA	NA	100–300	NA		NA
Polymethyl-methacrylate	Bone cement	25	NA	2	5	80		< 14
Cortical bone		80–160	NA	20	1–3	130–280	200–300	30

Vickers hardness is measured using a pyramidal indenter. The results have the dimensions of stress, and are usually expressed as kilograms force per square millimetre, but are here expressed as meganewtons per square metre for ease of comparison with the other properties. (Expressed in kgf/mm², the numerical values would be approximately one-tenth of those in the Table.)
  Strengths and stresses are given in meganewtons per square metre (i.e. 10^6 newtons per square metre), abbreviated to MN/m².
  Young's modulus has the dimensions of stress, and is given in giganewtons per square metre (i.e. 10^9 newtons per square metre), abbreviated to GN/m².
  The compressive strengths of metals and alloys are not given because they are not usually measured separately, being roughly equal to the respective ultimate tensile strengths.
  The tensile yield stress of aluminium oxide ceramic is not given because this is a brittle material and does not yield.
  'NA' in a space means that information is not available.
  The hardnesses of plastics are not readily measured by indentation methods; the values obtained by the methods which are used are equivalent to values in the range 50–200 MN/m².
  The properties given in this Table, and throughout the book, are expressed in units of the Système Internationale (SI). The following are the units chiefly used.
Mass: the kilogram (kg), equal to 1000 grams or 2·2 pounds.
Force: the newton (N), equal to 0·225 pounds force.
Length: the metre (m), equal to 39·36 inches.
         the millimetre (mm), 10^{-3} metre.
         the micrometre (μm), 10^{-6} metre, equal to 39·36 microinches.
Stress: newtons per square metre (N/m²) or, more usually, 10^6 newtons per square metre (meganewtons per square metre, MN/m²).

2.3 Fatigue

Figure 1.6.
The fatigue-fracture surface of a Charnley femoral stem (showing initiation site on lateral surface).

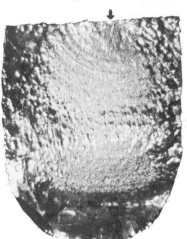

As previously discussed, the static mechanical properties of polymeric materials prevent their use in highly stressed components. While ceramic materials can withstand large static compressive stresses, their brittleness precludes them from use in situations where tensile stresses are likely to be encountered (for example, the intramedullary stems of total hip replacement femoral components; see Chapter 2, section 3.2).

As Table 1.1 shows, the available data indicate that annealed stainless steel, cast cobalt–chromium alloy, and titanium have similar fatigue resistance when tested in air.

Although fatigue has not been a major problem with total joint replacement components in the past, the incidence of femoral stem fatigue fractures in total hip prostheses (Fig. 1.6) now appears to be increasing, and fatigue may become a major cause of late failure in the future. Charnley's figures for his own total hip illustrate the point: there was only 1 stem fracture up to 1971 (Charnley 1971), there were 6 by 1973 (Charnley 1973) and 17 by 1975 (Charnley 1975), at periods from $1\frac{1}{2}$ to 6 years after operation. In this latest paper Charnley reported that whereas his over-all fracture rate was only 0.23 per cent, the rate for males having a body mass over 88 kg was 6.0 per cent. The predominant cause of fracture was thought to be lack of support to the proximal stem due to resorption of the calcar femorale.

Galante, Rostoker and Doyle (1975) examined six fractured femoral stems: four cast cobalt–chromium alloy Müller prostheses, and two stainless steel Charnley prostheses. A third Charnley fracture was mentioned but this had not been removed from the patient and so could not be examined. Six of the stems had fractured within two years while the seventh had lasted just over three years. All the fracture surfaces examined exhibited fatigue striations. Factors contributing to fatigue failure were identified as varus positioning and loosening of the stems, both of which would produce increased stress levels, and metallurgical defects.

Markolf and Amstutz (1976) studied three femoral stem failures. Metallurgical examination of a cast cobalt–chromium Müller prosthesis which had fractured 16 months after insertion showed fracture surface markings typical of fatigue but no obvious material defects. A stainless steel Bechtol stem showed gross plastic deformation in the proximal region but had not fractured. A second stainless steel Bechtol stem had yielded and fractured, the fracture being attributed to fatigue. Markolf and Amstutz mentioned two other fractured stems but did not give details.

There are two ways in which the technologist can help to reduce the incidence of femoral stem fatigue fractures: (1) by introducing new materials with increased fatigue strength; and (2) by redesigning the stems so as to reduce the magnitude of the stresses produced in them.

Other metals with significantly higher fatigue strengths in air than stainless steel, cast cobalt–chromium alloy and titanium include a cobalt–chromium-based, tungsten–nickel-alloyed material (so-called wrought cobalt–chromium alloy), a cobalt–nickel-based, chromium–molybdenum–titanium-alloyed material (MP 35 N or Protasul-10), and titanium alloyed with aluminium and vanadium. On the basis of a limited amount of corrosion data (see next section) the titanium alloy appears to offer the best promise for the future. (The wear performance of the alloy is uncertain but this potential problem can be overcome by combining cast cobalt–chromium alloy and titanium alloy in the same component. This combination does not produce galvanic corrosion because both alloys remain passivated.)

As Fig. 1.6 illustrates, the fatigue fracture of femoral stems is initiated by the tensile stresses produced on the lateral surface by the bending action of the load across the joint. Various design changes which could reduce the magnitude of these stresses are considered in Chapter 2.

2.4 Corrosion

Annealed stainless steel, cast cobalt–chromium alloy and titanium all exhibit passivity. However, laboratory tests on isolated specimens in physiological fluids (Hoar and Mears 1966) have shown that breakdown of the passivation film and pitting after long periods in the body are likely for annealed stainless steel, scarcely possible for cast cobalt–chromium alloy, and impossible for titanium.

Although the literature contains many reports of a high incidence of crevice corrosion in stainless steel implants, distinctions have to be made between types of implant and types of stainless steel. The majority of reported cases have been of crevice corrosion in multi-component stainless steel implants such as bone plates and screws (for example, Colangelo and Greene 1969). The crevices formed between screwhead and plate and any relative motion between them make this type of implant inherently more susceptible to crevice corrosion than the one-piece components of total joint replacements (see section 1.5 of this chapter). Also, the majority of multi-component stainless steel implants are manufactured in the cold-worked alloy for high strength whereas total joint components are usually made of annealed stainless steel for greater corrosion resistance (Semlitsch 1974). In practice the incidence of corrosion in stainless steel total joint replacement components is low. As far as the present author is aware the only report is that of Charnley (1971) in which he found that 18 out of 133 hips (15 per cent) removed because of the use of polytetrafluorethylene (PTFE) for the acetabular component appeared to show some corrosion. Even this incidence of corrosion is probably misleadingly high since more recent changes in the composition of surgical grade stainless steel (particularly a reduction in carbon content to a maximum of 0.03 per cent) have increased the corrosion resistance of the material.

No cases of corrosion of either cast cobalt–chromium alloy or titanium total joint replacement components have been reported.

Since the excellent fatigue resistance of wrought cobalt–chromium alloy, the cobalt–nickel-based alloy, and titanium alloyed with aluminium and vanadium suggest these materials for use in total joint replacements, their corrosion resistance must be considered. While wrought cobalt–chromium alloy is now widely used for other types of orthopaedic implant (for example, bone plates and hip pins and plates), Cohen and Wulff (1972) have reported a case of crevice corrosion in such an implant, and shown in the laboratory that the wrought alloy is more susceptible to crevice corrosion than the cast alloy.

Although the cobalt–nickel-based alloy (MP 35 N) has been used for certain total joint replacements since 1971 (Semlitsch 1974), the corrosion data on the material appear to be contradictory. After laboratory tests, Süry (1974) concluded that the alloy has even higher resistance to pitting and crevice corrosion in chloride-containing media than cast cobalt–chromium alloy, while Devine and Wulff (1975) found that resistance to crevice corrosion increased in the order stainless steel, MP 35 N, wrought cobalt–chromium alloy, cast cobalt–chromium alloy.

The laboratory findings of Hoar and Mears (1966) indicate that titanium alloys, like pure titanium, should be even more corrosion resistant in the body than cast cobalt–chromium alloy.

Polymers and ceramics cannot corrode but they can be degraded chemically by their environment. Table 1.1 lists four polymeric materials which are, or have been, used to provide one of the bearing surfaces in total joint replacements. Of these, high molecular weight polyethylene has proved to be the most successful, principally because of its high resistance to degradation. Nylon 66 readily absorbs water and this rapidly reduces its tensile strength in the human body (Williams 1971). Although the water absorption of polyester is relatively low, laboratory tests have shown it to be degraded by hydrolysis (Scales 1972), and a total hip replacement consisting of a polyester ball in a metal cup failed due to excess polymer wear, presumably resulting from degradation (Weber and Stühmer 1976; and see Chapter 3, section 2.4). Delrin, a polyacetal, is currently in use in one particular design of total hip replacement, with apparent success (Sundal, Kavlie and Christiansen 1974), but the material has a relatively high water absorption (Williams 1971) and its long-term stability in the body has yet to be demonstrated.

Although there are many references in the literature to the chemical inertness of aluminium oxide ceramic and several total hip replacements with aluminium oxide bearing surfaces are in current use (see, for example, Boutin 1972), Schmittgrund, Kenner and Brown (1973) state that the material loses strength when left unstressed in saline solution, or in the soft tissues of dogs or rabbits. The same authors found that another ceramic proposed for use as an implant material, calcium aluminate, also lost strength when soaked in saline or implanted *in vivo*.

2.5 Corrosion-fatigue

Although the reported incidence of corrosion of stainless steel joint components is low and corrosion alone has never produced mechanical failure of such components, corrosion-fatigue must be a possibility. Charnley, reporting on the use of stainless steel in total hip prostheses in 1971, stated that high corrosion-fatigue resistance is perhaps more important than high fatigue resistance in materials for permanent implants. In the same paper Charnley reported that the only fracture in the stainless steel component of his hip prosthesis (to that date) had been ascribed to corrosion-fatigue, fracture having been initiated at a corrosion pit.

Colangelo (1969) conducted laboratory fatigue tests on notched specimens of annealed surgical stainless steel in air and saline. Crack propagation was faster in saline solution than in air and there was a distinct difference in the appearance of the fracture surfaces. Specimens broken in air had a bright, lustrous appearance while those broken in saline had a dull fracture surface darkened with corrosion products. Colangelo concluded that corrosion could accelerate crack propagation as well as crack initiation in this material.

Although only one of the femoral stem fractures so far reported in the literature has been attributed to corrosion-fatigue rather than pure fatigue, it seems likely that corrosion has played a part in the fracture of at least some of the stainless steel stems. In cases where one of the factors contributing to fracture has been the breakdown of cement fixation in the proximal half of the stem, a situation likely to produce crevice corrosion would seem to exist. The breakdown of the metal–cement bond may produce a long narrow crevice with low oxygen concentration, and any relative motion between stem and cement could lead to the abrasive removal of the passivating film.

Of the higher fatigue strength materials, only wrought cobalt–chromium alloy has been shown to be susceptible to corrosion-fatigue in the body. Rose, Schiller and Radin (1972) examined a McLaughlin nail and plate, the plate of which had fractured immediately adjacent to the nail hole. Visual examination showed that the fracture had been initiated at the inner (bone) face where the nail teeth were in contact with the plate. Chemical analysis showed that the plate was wrought cobalt–chromium alloy whereas the nail was made of the cast alloy. Since wrought cobalt–chromium alloy is normally a fairly ductile material, the lack of any appreciable gross plastic deformation of the plate indicated fatigue failure. However, fracture had been initiated from a site normally in compression, and the fracture surface had the appearance of a brittle fracture with none of the characteristics of a fatigue fracture in a ductile material. That is, there were no microslip lines on the surface of the plate, there was no shear lip, and there were no fatigue striations. Scanning electron microscopy showed cleavage steps indicative of brittle fracture on the fracture surface, and microcracks leading from pits on the surface of the plate. The authors concluded that fracture initiation had been assisted by corrosion and that this process changed the mechanism of crack propagation from a normally ductile mode to a brittle mode. In support of this conclusion the paper included scanning electron micrographs of the fracture surface of wrought cobalt–chromium alloy specimens fatigue tested in air. These control specimens showed the characteristic features of fatigue fracture in ductile materials, including fatigue striations.

The chemical degradation of polymers and ceramics in certain environments can be accelerated by fluctuating stress. It seems likely that this degradative fatigue process was at least partly responsible for the excessively high wear rate of polytetrafluorethylene and polyester in total hip replacements, and there is evidence to suggest that it also plays a part in the wear of high molecular weight polyethylene (see Chapter 3, section 2.3).

As mentioned in the previous section, Schmittgrund, Kenner and Brown (1973) found that aluminium oxide ceramic degrades when soaked in saline and the soft tissues of animals. The same authors state that the material exhibits a significant loss of strength in a moist air environment if subjected to a cyclic stress in excess of 112 MN/m^2.

2.6 Summary

Only metallic materials have the static tensile strength and fatigue resistance required for the highly stressed parts of total joint replacements. The added requirements of high corrosion and corrosion-fatigue resistance restrict the choice of metals and alloys to surgical grade stainless steel, cast cobalt–chromium alloy, chromium–nickel alloy, titanium, and titanium alloyed with aluminium and vanadium. Of these, the last appears to offer the best combination of mechanical and electrochemical properties. The wear performance of the alloy might be a problem, but this can be overcome by using cast cobalt–chromium for the bearing surface.

Polymers are inherently weak materials and consequently cannot be used in high stress situations. Their use as bearing materials in total joint replacements (low stress conditions) is based on their low friction against metals and the fact that some polymeric wear debris appears to be better tolerated by the body than metallic wear debris (see Chapter 4). As far as the mechanical properties are concerned, the major problem with the use of polymers as bearing materials in the body is degradation. Nylon 66 and polyethylene terephthalate (a polyester) have proved unsuccessful and the long-term stability of Delrin (a polyacetal) in the body has yet to be demonstrated. High molecular weight polyethylene has proved to be the most successful polymer and is now widely used to provide one of the bearing surfaces of total joint replacements. The friction and wear of polymeric materials and the effects of degradation are discussed in Chapter 3.

Ceramic materials are extremely brittle and therefore cannot be used in situations where high tensile stresses are produced. They are, however, extremely strong in compression, extremely hard, and generally inert. A total hip replacement with aluminium oxide bearing surfaces has apparently proved successful over a number of years but there is some evidence that the material may degrade in the body. Information about the wear resistance of the material is both limited and contradictory, but this is discussed in more detail in Chapter 3.

BIBLIOGRAPHY

Implants in Surgery. (1973) D. F. Williams and R. Roaf. Philadelphia, Pa., and London, W. B. Saunders.

An Introduction to Orthopædic Materials. (1975) J. H. Dumbleton and J. Black. Springfield, Ill., Charles C Thomas.

The Structure and Properties of Materials. Vol. II, *Thermodynamics of Structure.* (1964) J. H. Brophy, R. M. Rose and J. Wulff. New York and Chichester, John Wiley.

The Structure and Properties of Materials. Vol. III, *Mechanical Behaviour.* (1965) H. W. Hayden, W. G. Moffatt and J. Wulff. New York and Chichester, John Wiley.

REFERENCES

Boutin, P. (1972) Arthroplastie totale de la hanche par prothèse en alumine frittée. *Revue de Chirurgie Orthopédique et Réparatrice de l'Appareil Moteur* **58**, 229.

Charnley, J. (1971) Stainless steel for femoral hip prostheses in combination with a high density polythene socket. *Journal of Bone and Joint Surgery* **53B**, 342.

Charnley, J. (1973) Biomechanical considerations in total hip prosthetic design. In, *The Hip*. St Louis, Mo., C. V. Mosby.

Charnley, J. (1975) Fracture of femoral prostheses in total hip replacement. A clinical study. *Clinical Orthopaedics and Related Research* **111**, 105.

Cohen, J. and Wulff, J. (1972) Clinical fracture caused by corrosion of a vitallium plate. *Journal of Bone and Joint Surgery* **54A**, 617.

Colangelo, V. J. (1969) Corrosion fatigue in surgical implants. *Journal of Basic Engineering (Trans. ASME)* December, 581.

Colangelo, V. J. and Greene, N. D. (1969) Corrosion and fracture of Type 316 SMO orthopaedic implants. *Journal of Biomedical Materials Research* **3**, 247.

Devine, T. M. and Wulff, J. (1975) Cast vs. wrought cobalt–chromium surgical implant alloys. *Journal of Biomedical Materials Research* **9**, 151.

Galante, J. O., Rostoker, W. and Doyle, J. M. (1975) Failed femoral stems in total hip prostheses. *Journal of Bone and Joint Surgery* **57A**, 230.

Hoar, T. P. and Mears, D. C. (1966) Corrosion-resistant alloys in chloride solutions: materials for surgical implants. *Proceedings of the Royal Society*, **A294**, 486.

Markolf, K. and Amstutz, H. (1976) A comparative experimental study of stresses in femoral total hip replacement components: the effects of prosthesis orientation and acrylic fixation. *Journal of Biomechanics* **9**, 73.

Rose, R. M., Schiller, A. L. and Radin, E. L. (1972) Corrosion-accelerated mechanical failure of a Vitallium nail-plate. *Journal of Bone and Joint Surgery* **54A**, 854.

Scales, J. T. (1972) Some aspects of Stanmore total hip prostheses and their development. In, *Arthroplasty of the Hip*, p. 113. Ed. G. Chapchal. Stuttgart, Thieme.

Schmittgrund, G. D., Kenner, G. H. and Brown S. D. (1973) In vivo and in vitro changes in strength of orthopaedic calcium aluminates. *Journal of Biomedical Materials Research, Symposium No. 4*, 435.

Semlitsch, M. (1974) Technical progress in artificial hip joints. *Sulzer Review* **4**.

Sundal, B., Kavlie, H. and Christiansen, T. (1974) Total hip replacement with a new trunnion-bearing prosthesis (the Christiansen prosthesis). *Acta Chirurgica Scandinavica* **140**, 189.

Süry, P. (1974) Corrosion behaviour of cast and forged implant material for artificial joints particularly with respect to compound designs. *Sulzer Research*.

Weber, G. G. and Stühmer, G. (1976) Experience with trunnion bearing prosthesis with head of polyester material. In, International Symposium on Advances in Artificial Hip and Knee Joint Technology, Erlangen, W. Germany. *Engineering in Medicine*. Berlin, Springer-Verlag. In the press.

Williams, D. F. (1971) The properties and medical uses of materials, Part 5. *Biomedical Engineering* **6**, 300.

CHAPTER TWO

Stress Analysis

1 BASIC THEORY

1.1 Tension and Compression

THE internal stresses produced in a prismatic bar loaded in simple (uniaxial) tension (Fig 2.1a) can be analysed by imagining the bar cut into pieces along various planes.

If the bar were to be cut on planes at right angles to the direction of loading the lower part would move downwards under the action of the externally applied force, F. Since this does not happen in the uncut bar, the external force must be balanced by an equal force acting upwards on the section. Similarly there must be an equal force acting downwards on the upper part of the bar (Fig. 2.1b). These two forces represent the action of each part of the bar on the other.

The average tensile stress, defined as the ratio of force to area, acting on the section is equal to F/A (Fig. 2.1c), and if the internal forces are evenly distributed over the cross-section the stresses at all points will be equal to this average stress. Clearly, the situation is the same for all planes at right angles to the direction of loading.

The situation is more complex on planes inclined to the load axis (Fig. 2.1d). Each part of the bar is again in equilibrium under the combined action of external forces and internal stresses (Fig. 2.1e) but the internal stresses are no longer normal to the plane of the section. If the stresses are resolved (split) into components acting normally and tangentially to the section (Fig. 2.1f), it can be seen that the two parts of the bar are tending to separate under the action of the normal components and to slip, or shear, relative to each other under the action of the tangential, or shear, component.

All planes through the bar can be described by this general case of an inclined plane, simply by varying the angle of the plane. That is, the stresses acting on any plane consist of a normal stress and a shear stress, the magnitudes of each depending on the angle of the plane to the load axis. Planes at right angles and at 45° to the load axis are of particular interest because the normal stress has a maximum value on the former while the shear stress has a maximum value on the latter. Since the maximum value of shear stress is only one-half the maximum value of normal stress, all materials might be expected to

Figure 2.1.
Uniaxial tension.

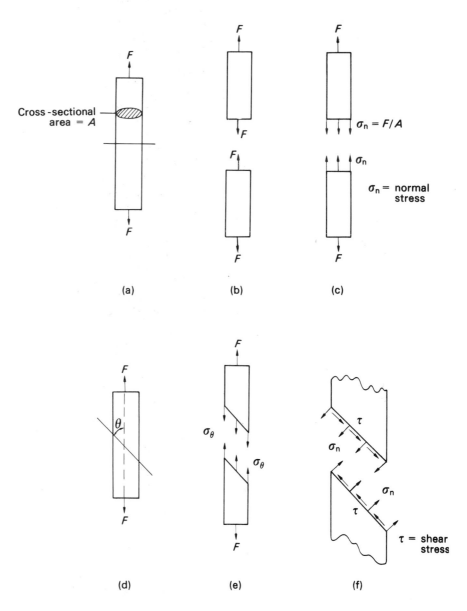

fracture on planes at right angles to the load axis in simple tension. Some materials, however, whose shear strength is less than half their tensile strength, fracture by a shearing process on planes at 45° to the load axis.

One other aspect of simple tension, the deformation produced, should be considered. The externally applied tensile force produces both an axial extension and a lateral contraction of the bar, the magnitudes of which depend on the magnitude of the applied stress and the material of the bar.

For most materials the ratio of the applied tensile stress to the axial extension per unit length (axial strain) is found to be a constant up to a certain level of stress (see Chapter 1). This constant is called the tension modulus, or Young's modulus (E), of the material, so that

$$E = \frac{\text{tensile stress } (\sigma_x)}{\text{axial strain } (e_x)}$$

where $\sigma_x = F/A$, and

$$e_x = \frac{\text{extension}}{\text{original length}}$$

The unit lateral contraction (lateral strain) is found to be related to the axial strain by another material constant called Poisson's ratio (ν), so that

$$\nu = \frac{\text{lateral strain } (e_x)}{\text{axial strain } (e_y)}$$

The above analysis of simple tension applies also to uniaxial compression, the only difference being that by convention tensile stresses are taken as positive and compressive stresses negative.

1.2 Pure Bending

A simple beam subjected to bending (Fig. 2.2a) will deform as in Fig. 2.2b. Longitudinal elements on the convex side of the beam are elongated (a–b going to a′–b′) whereas similar elements on the concave side are compressed (c–d going to c′–d′). Between these two extremes there is a position at which the length of longitudinal elements is unchanged during bending and this is the so-called neutral axis (NA) of the beam.

Since the internal stresses produced are directly proportional to the strains, the stress distribution over any cross-section of the beam is as shown in Fig. 2.2c. Compressive stresses are produced on the concave side and tensile stresses on the convex side, the magnitude of both increasing linearly with distance from the neutral axis. The combined effect of these tensile and compressive stresses is to provide a moment or torque on the section to balance the externally applied bending moment at the free end.

Analysis shows that the magnitude of the stresses produced by bending is given by

$$\sigma = \frac{M.y}{I_F}$$

where M is the externally applied bending moment,

y is the distance from the neutral axis, and

I_F is the flexural second moment of area of the beam cross-section.

(The second moment of area of a cross-section is a quantitative measure of the way in which the cross-sectional area is distributed about a particular axis. In bending the relevant axis is the axis in the plane of the cross-section, perpendicular to the plane of the diagram in Fig 2.2, and passing through the centre of gravity of the cross-section, and the second moment of area about this axis is known as the flexural second moment of area.)

Figure 2.2.
Pure bending.

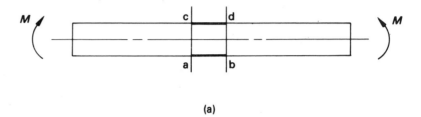

(a)

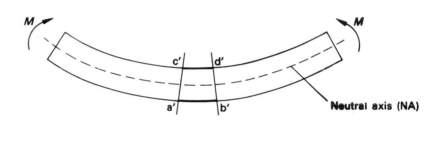

(b)

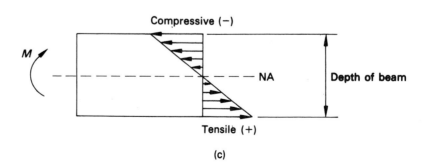

(c)

The maximum bending stresses are produced at the top (compressive) and bottom (tensile) surfaces of the beam and their magnitude is given by

$$\sigma_{max} = \frac{M.d}{2I_F}$$

where d is the depth of the beam.

A large second moment of area (I_F) means that the stresses, and the corresponding strains, are lower for a given applied bending moment (M) and depth of cross-section (d) than if I_F is smaller. Thus a beam having a high value of I_F is both stronger and stiffer in bending than one having a lower value of I_F. For example, the flexural second moment of area of I-section beams is high because a high proportion of the cross-sectional area is a large distance away from the neutral axis, and this is why they are used widely in civil engineering structures.

1.3 Combined Bending and Shear

Pure bending rarely occurs in practice; in most real situations bending and other types of loading occur simultaneously. A common example of this is a beam supported at both ends and loaded at its centre (Fig. 2.3a).

Consider a section A–A through the beam at right angles to its long axis. The part of the beam to the left of this section must be in equilibrium under the combined action of the force from the support and the internal stresses on the section. The force from the support is tending to rotate the left-hand part of the beam clockwise about the section and also to move it vertically upwards relative to the right-hand part. The turning effect is balanced by a bending moment at the section and the vertical motion is prevented by forces acting vertically downwards over the section (Fig. 2.3b). The bending moment produces tensile and compressive stresses just as in pure bending, while the forces acting downwards along the section produce shear stresses.

Shear stresses are also produced on longitudinal planes within the beam. If the beam were cut horizontally and then loaded it would deform as shown in Fig. 2.3c. Relative slipping would occur between the two parts of the beam along the cut surface. Since this does not occur in the uncut beam, shear forces and therefore shear stresses must be developed to prevent it.

Three-point bending differs from pure bending not only in the presence of shear forces but also in that the bending moment at sections of the beam varies with the position of the section along the beam. At section B–B in Fig. 2.3b, for example, the bending moment is given by

$$M_{BB} = \frac{L}{2}.x$$

where x is the distance of the section from the support.

This is because the bending moment at the section must balance the turning effect of the externally applied force and this is equal to the product of force and the moment arm of the force about the section. Figure 2.3d is a graph, the bending moment diagram, showing how the magnitude of the bending moment varies along the beam. Since the bending stresses produced in the beam are proportional to the bending moment, which is at its maximum at the centre of the beam, the maximum bending stresses in three-point bending are produced at that section.

Figure 2.3.
Bending and shear in three-point bending.

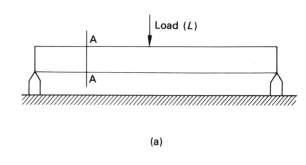

(a)

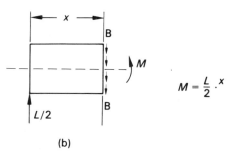

$$M = \frac{L}{2} \cdot x$$

(b)

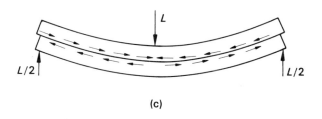

(c)

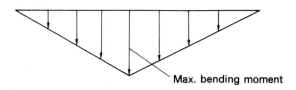

Max. bending moment

(d) Bending moment diagram

1.4 Combined Bending and Compression

Another example of bending combined with other forms of loading is provided by the case of a bar loaded axially in compression (or tension), but with the compressive forces displaced from the centre line of the bar (Fig. 2.4a).

Figure 2.4.
Combined bending and compression.

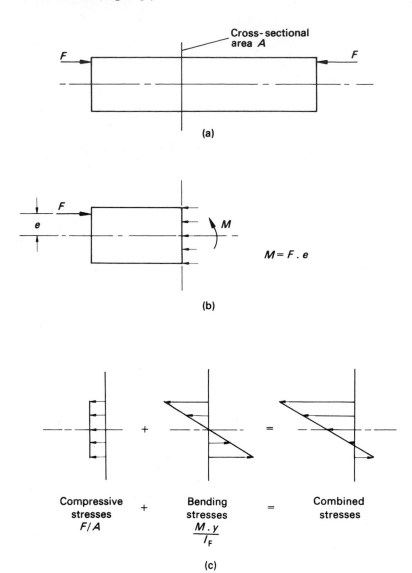

If the bar were cut at right angles to the direction of loading, the part on the left would try to move to the right and rotate under the action of the externally applied force. As in the previous examples, these motions are prevented in the uncut bar by internal stresses produced at the section (Fig. 2.4b). The horizontal motion is prevented by horizontal compressive stresses acting normal to the section, and the turning motion is prevented by a bending moment. The compressive stresses are equal to F/A, while the bending moment produces tensile and compressive bending stresses, the magnitudes of which depend on the bending moment at each section. In this case the bending moment is the same for all sections through the bar, and is given by

$$M = F.e$$

where e is the eccentricity or offset of the externally applied load from the centre line of the bar.

Because the compressive stresses and the bending stresses are in the same direction they can be added together to show the combined stress distribution across any section of the bar (Fig. 2.4c).

1.5 Torsion

Consider a solid circular shaft twisted about its axis (Fig. 2.5a). If the shaft were cut into two parts on a plane at right angles to its axis, the two parts would revolve freely in opposite directions under the action of the externally applied twisting moments (torques). In the uncut shaft this motion is prevented by internal stresses which provide equal and opposite turning moments (Fig. 2.5b). These stresses are shear stresses since they act tangentially over the cross-section.

As the shaft deforms (Fig. 2.5c), points on any radial line OA move to new positions along a new radial line OA'. The amount of deformation is therefore proportional to distance from the axis of the shaft. Just as in tension, the ratio of stress to strain in shear is a material constant, known as the shear modulus, G (equal to the ratio of shear stress to shear strain), so that the shear stress distribution over the cross-section (Fig. 2.5d) has the same shape as the strain distribution. The magnitude of the shear stress at any distance (r) from the shaft axis can be shown to be

$$\tau = \frac{M.r}{I_P}$$

where M is the twisting moment, or torque, and

I_P is the polar second moment of area of the cross-section about the axis of the shaft, a quantity of the same kind as the flexural second moment of area defined in section 1.2 above, but related to the axis of the shaft itself instead of to an axis perpendicular to it.

Since the maximum shear stress is produced at the outer surface of the shaft

$$\tau_{max} = \frac{M.D}{2I_P}$$

where D is the diameter of the shaft.

On any plane inclined to the axis of the shaft the internal forces preventing rotation can be resolved into components normal and tangential to the plane. (This is equivalent to the situation on inclined planes in uniaxial tension.) In general, therefore, there are normal stresses and shear stresses on all planes through the shaft. On planes parallel to and at right angles to the shaft axis the shear stresses are a maximum and the normal stresses are zero while on planes at 45° to the axis the normal stresses are a maximum and the shear stresses are zero (Fig. 2.5e). This explains why a shaft of brittle material, for example a stick of chalk, will fracture on planes at 45° to its axis when twisted: the material is failing in tension due to the normal tensile stresses produced on this plane.

In a solid circular shaft, material towards the centre is stressed to a lower level than material at the outside (Fig. 2.5d). Since the moment arm is also less towards the centre, material here is playing a relatively small part in resisting the applied torque. The fact that material is used more efficiently the greater its distance from the axis of the shaft explains why hollow shafts are used to resist torsion when weight is important.

Figure 2.5.
Torsion.

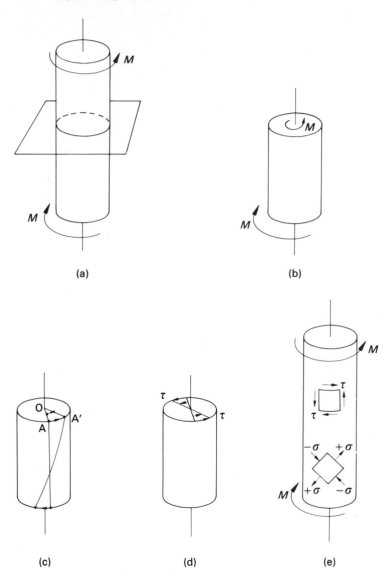

1.6 Composite Structures

Different materials are often combined in engineering components subjected to load, and it is important to be able to calculate the stresses produced in each material.

1.6.1 COMPRESSION

Consider the case of a solid circular cylinder of one material inside a circular tube of another material, the combined structure being compressed between two rigid plates as shown in Fig. 2.6a. The applied compressive force is carried partly by the cylinder and partly by the tube (Fig. 2.6b), so that

$$F = F_C + F_T$$

where F_C is the force on the cylinder, and
F_T is the force on the tube.

If the compressive stress on the cylinder is σ_C and the Young's modulus of the cylinder material is E_C, then the strain of the cylinder (e_C) is given by

$$e_C = \frac{\sigma_C}{E_C}$$

Similarly, if the compressive stress on the tube is σ_T and the Young's modulus of the tube material is E_T, the strain of the tube (e_T) is given by

$$e_T = \frac{\sigma_T}{E_T}$$

Since the cylinder and tube were originally the same length and they are compressed by the same amount, the strain of the cylinder is equal to the strain of the tube.

That is,

$$\frac{\sigma_C}{E_C} = \frac{\sigma_T}{E_T}$$

or

$$\frac{\sigma_C}{\sigma_T} = \frac{E_C}{E_T}$$

Thus, the ratio of the stresses produced in the cylinder and the tube is the same as the ratio of the Young's moduli of the two materials (Fig. 2.6c).

Since stress is equal to force divided by area, the last expression can be rewritten to give

$$\frac{F_C}{F_T} = \frac{E_C A_C}{E_T A_T}$$

The effective stiffness of a structure in compression (i.e. the amount of deformation produced by a given compressive force) depends on the intrinsic stiffness of the material (E) and the cross-sectional area of the structure. The equation above therefore shows that the applied compressive force is divided between the two component structures in proportion to their compressive stiffnesses; that is, the stiffer component carries a higher proportion of the load.

Figure 2.6.
Compression of a composite structure.

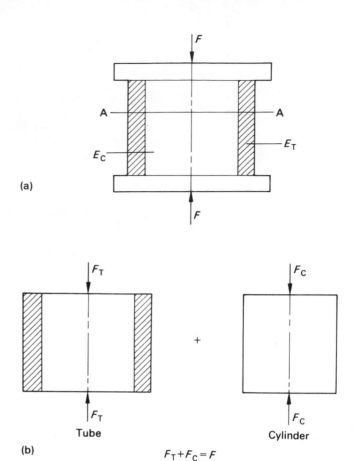

(a)

(b)

$$F_T + F_C = F$$

Tube   Cylinder

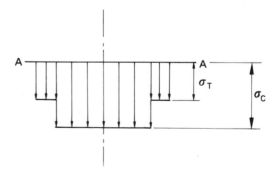

(c) Compressive stress distribution ($E_T < E_C$)

Figure 2.7a shows a rectangular section beam of one material with plates of another material fixed to the top and bottom surfaces. If the **composite** structure is subjected to pure bending, the applied bending moment is carried partly by the beam and partly by the plates (Fig. 2.7b), so that

$$M = M_B + M_P$$

where M is the applied bending moment,

M_B is the bending moment carried by the beam, and

M_P is the bending moment carried by the plates.

If the bending stress produced on the outer surfaces of the beam is denoted by σ_B, then, since

$$\sigma = \frac{M.y}{I_F},$$

$$\sigma_B = \frac{M_B.d}{2I_{FB}}$$

where d is the depth of the beam, and

I_{FB} is the flexural second moment of area of the beam cross-section.

Figure 2.7.
Bending of a composite beam.

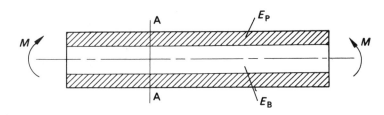

(a)

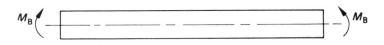

$$M_B + M_P = M$$

(b)

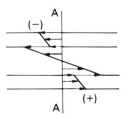

(c) Bending stress distribution ($E_P < E_B$)

If the bending stress on the inner surface of the plates is σ_P, then

$$\sigma_P = \frac{M_P.d}{2I_{FP}}$$

Since the strains in the beam and plates at the interface must be the same, the ratio of the stresses there must be the same as the ratio of the Young's moduli. That is,

$$\frac{\sigma_B}{\sigma_P} = \frac{E_B}{E_P}$$

Thus the bending stress distribution over a cross-section of the composite structure when the Young's modulus of the plate material is less than that of the beam material is as shown in Fig. 2.7c.

Substituting the expressions for each stress into the above equation gives

$$\frac{M_B}{M_P} = \frac{E_B.I_{FB}}{E_P.I_{FP}}$$

The stiffness of a structure in bending is made up of two factors, the stiffness of the material (E) and the resistance to bending offered by the cross-sectional shape of the structure (I_F), and the product (EI_F) is therefore called flexural rigidity or bending stiffness. The importance of the last equation is that it shows that in a composite beam subjected to bending the applied bending moment is divided between the two components of the structure in proportion to their bending stiffnesses.

1.6.3 TORSION

A composite shaft subjected to torsion (Fig. 2.8) is exactly equivalent to a composite beam in bending. That is, since the strains in the two materials at the interface are the same, the shear stresses there are in proportion to the shear moduli, and the proportions of the applied torque carried by the two components depend on their respective torsional rigidities. Expressed mathematically,

$$\frac{\tau_C}{\tau_T} = \frac{G_C}{G_T}$$

$$M = M_C + M_T$$

and

$$\frac{M_C}{M_T} = \frac{G_C.I_{PC}}{G_T.I_{PT}}$$

where τ_C and τ_T are the shear stresses at the interface in the cylinder and tube respectively,

G_C and G_T are the shear moduli of cylinder and tube materials,

M is the applied torque,

M_C and M_T are the torques carried by the cylinder and tube, and

I_{PC} and I_{PT} are the polar second moments of area of the cylinder and tube.

Figure 2.8.
Torsion of a composite shaft.

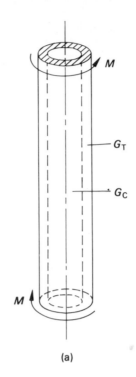

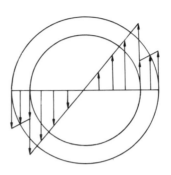

(b) Shear stress distribution ($G_T < G_C$)

(a)

1.7 Summary

1.7.1 UNIAXIAL TENSION (OR COMPRESSION)

On any plane inclined to the load axis uniaxial loading produces tensile or compressive stresses and shear stresses, the magnitudes of which vary with the angle of inclination of the plane. The tensile or compressive stresses are at a maximum on planes at right angles to the load axis and the shear stresses are at a maximum on planes at 45° to the load axis.

The maximum average tensile or compressive stress is given by

$$\sigma = F/A$$

where F is the applied load, and
A is the cross-sectional area of the component.

1.7.2 PURE BENDING

Subjecting a beam to pure bending produces stresses which vary linearly over any cross-section from a maximum tensile stress at one surface to a maximum compressive stress at the opposite surface.

The value of these maximum stresses is directly proportional to the applied bending moment and the depth of the beam and inversely proportional to the flexural second moment of area of the cross-sectional shape. That is,

$$\sigma_{\max} = \frac{M.d}{2I_F}$$

where M is the applied bending moment,
d is the depth of the beam, and
I_F is the flexural second moment of area of the beam cross-section.

31

1.7.3 TORSION

Subjecting a shaft to torsion produces shear stresses and normal stresses (tension and compression) on any plane inclined to the shaft axis. On planes at right angles to the shaft axis, where the normal stresses are zero, the maximum shear stress is produced at the surface of the shaft and has a magnitude proportional to the torque being applied and the diameter of the shaft and inversely proportional to the polar second moment of area of the shaft cross-section. That is,

$$\tau_{max} = \frac{M.D}{2I_P}$$

where M is the applied torque,
D is the diameter of the shaft, and
I_P is the polar second moment of area of the cross-section.

Maximum normal stresses are produced on planes inclined at 45° to the shaft axis.

1.7.4 COMBINED LOADING

Structures are rarely subjected to only one type of loading. However, it is often possible to analyse the nature and magnitudes of the stresses produced by a complex form of loading by treating it as a combination of different types of simple loading. Eccentric compression, for example, can be treated as a combination of uniaxial compression and pure bending.

1.7.5 COMPOSITE STRUCTURES

In most cases it is extremely difficult to analyse the stresses produced in the different elements of a composite structure, since any such analysis requires some knowledge of the deformation of the structure. However, the analysis of simple composite structures subjected to simple loading shows that, in general, the applied loads are divided between the structural elements in proportion to their respective stiffnesses. That is:

(1) an applied compressive load is divided between the elements in proportion to their compressive stiffnesses ($E.A$);

(2) an applied bending moment is divided between the elements in proportion to their flexural stiffnesses ($E.I_F$); and

(3) an applied torque is divided between the elements in proportion to their torsional stiffnesses ($G.I_P$).

Once the individual loads on each structural element are known the stresses produced can be calculated.

For further study of basic stress analysis the reader is referred to the bibliography at the end of this chapter.

2 EXPERIMENTAL STRESS ANALYSIS

It is often impossible to calculate by simple theory the stresses produced in complex structures, and in these cases it becomes necessary to measure the stresses experimentally. Also, in many situations it is desirable to check calculated values by experiment. Although a detailed description of all the available experimental methods is beyond the scope of this book, a brief summary of three of the most frequently used techniques is given below.

2.1 Brittle Coatings

This technique consists of slowly loading a specimen after first coating its surface with a thin layer of a brittle material which will crack at a known tensile strain. Whenever a crack first appears, its position, direction and the load on the specimen at the time are noted. Since the coating is thin and firmly attached to the specimen, the strain in the coating is the same as in the surface of the specimen. Therefore, when a crack appears, the strain in the surface of the specimen at the position of the crack is known and the stress can be calculated using the Young's modulus of the specimen material. Since the coating cracks at right angles to the maximum tensile strain, the calculated stress is the maximum tensile stress at that point and its direction is known. The maximum tensile stress at this point under any other value of applied load is a matter of simple proportion since stress is directly proportional to load within the elastic range.

As the load on the specimen increases, more and more cracks appear. At the end of test the maximum tensile stress at each point where a crack appeared can be calculated for one fixed value of applied load to give the picture of the maximum tensile stress distribution over the entire specimen.

The maximum compressive stress distribution can be obtained by coating the specimen when loaded and then noting the position, direction and load at which cracks appear as the load is released. A complete picture of the surface stress field is therefore obtained from two relatively easy tests.

2.2 Strain Gauges

If a length of wire is strained, its electrical resistance changes. Since it is relatively easy to measure changes in resistance this behaviour forms the basis of a convenient method of measuring strain, and therefore stress.

The most common type of strain gauge consists of a grid of wire bonded to a paper backing. The gauge is cemented to the surface being studied so that its change in resistance as the specimen is loaded measures the strains (tensile or compressive) produced in the surface. Figure 2.9 shows strain gauges attached to the lateral surface of the stem of the femoral component of a hip prosthesis.

Because the electrical resistance of wire changes with temperature as well as strain, it is normal practice to arrange for temperature effects to be cancelled by a 'dummy' (unstrained) gauge maintained at the same temperature as the active gauge on a piece of similar material.

2.3 Photoelasticity

When polarised light is passed through a loaded sheet of a birefringent material and viewed through a polariser, two superimposed sets of stress patterns or fringes are produced. One of these patterns, the isoclinics, provides information about the direction of the maximum direct stress at various points; the other, the isochromatics, provides information about the difference between the maximum and minimum tensile or compressive stresses at various points. The stress distribution in a loaded structure can be obtained by making a model of the structure in a birefringent material and applying special techniques to analyse the fringe patterns. The technique as thus outlined is essentially two-dimensional, but a considerably more complicated three-dimensional technique is available. In either two- or three-dimensional form, photoelasticity produces information about the stresses in the photoelastic model, which is naturally homogeneous. The technique is thus of limited value for finding stresses in skeletal components, and for finding stresses in prosthetic components strain gauges are preferred because they can be attached to the components themselves instead of to models.

3 THE STRESS ANALYSIS OF TOTAL JOINT REPLACEMENTS

3.1 The Place of Theoretical and Experimental Stress Analysis

Ideally, a complete stress analysis of every design of total joint replacement should be carried out before clinical use to ensure that the stresses which will be produced *in vivo* will not produce failure. Unfortunately, this ideal is impractical for the following reasons:

(1) Any prosthetic joint component is stressed by a combination of forces and moments applied across the articulating surface and forces and moments applied across its interface with the bone (or cement). All these loads can vary in three dimensions and with time, and result partly from forces in muscles and ligaments which are difficult or impossible to ascertain.

(2) A total joint replacement component cemented into bone forms a composite structure of three materials. The complicated shape of the structure and the four-dimensional nature of the loading mean that (i) the stresses produced vary from point to point throughout the three materials, (ii) at each point the stresses consist of a combination of tensile or compressive stress and shear stress, and (iii) the magnitudes of the stresses at each point vary with time.

(3) Even if the magnitude of the stresses could be calculated from a knowledge or estimate of the applied loads and the elastic moduli of the three materials, it would still not be possible to predict with any certainty whether or not failure would occur. This is because the known fracture strengths of materials are obtained from laboratory tests under conditions of simple loading (e.g. tension only), and it is difficult to predict from these data what combinations of stress will produce fracture.

Thus, a combination of complexity and lack of data makes it impossible to design a perfect total joint replacement solely from theoretical considerations. While the use of computers and special analytical techniques such as finite element analysis can help to overcome the problem of complexity, even the most sophisticated

Figure 2.9.
Strain gauges attached to the lateral
surface of the stem of a hip prosthesis.

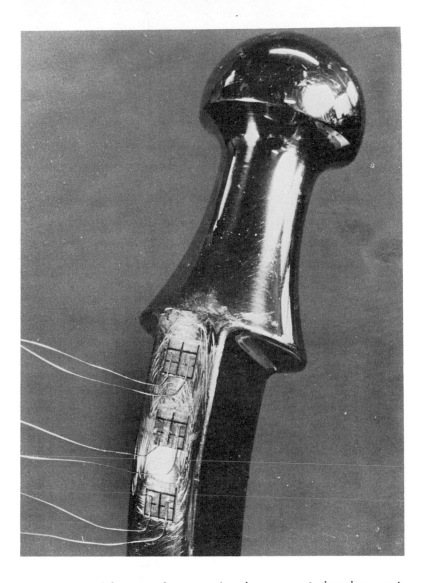

computer models are only approximations to real situations and, clearly, the use of a computer cannot solve the problem of lack of data. It follows that the development of successful joint replacements must involve a combination of simplified theoretical stress analysis, experimental stress analysis, laboratory testing, and clinical experience.

At the present time two different situations are of practical importance: the improvement of existing total joint replacements, and the development of entirely new ones. In the former case clinical experience will have highlighted a particular problem; for example, the occasional fracture of a prosthetic component. Examination of the failures will indicate a particular region of excessively high stress, and relatively simple theoretical stress analysis will suggest design changes which should reduce the stress. Finally, experimental stress analysis techniques can be used to confirm the reduction in stress before clinical use.

In the second case the new total joint replacement should be inserted into post-mortem joints and tested in the laboratory under, as far as possible, physiological loading conditions. Again, relatively simple stress analysis can be applied to any failure sites so as to improve the design. If the nature and magnitude of the physiological loading are unknown then the strength of post-mortem specimens fitted with the new prosthesis should be compared with specimens of the normal joint under various types of loading (e.g. compression, bending and torsion), and every effort should be made to produce an artificial joint which will not fail at lower loads than the natural joint. The new total joint replacement should be clinically tested only after such rigorous laboratory development. If clinical failure then occurs the development work should continue as described above.

In practice, total joint replacements fail in one of two ways to which stress analysis is directly relevant: they fracture or they loosen. The magnitudes of the stresses produced in the cement and bone around replacements are clearly an important factor in loosening, but since the mechanical aspects of fixation are considered in another part of this book (Chapter 5) the remainder of this chapter will concentrate on the role of theoretical and experimental stress analysis in preventing prosthesis fracture.

It is not possible in a book of this kind to discuss the stress analysis of every design of every type of total joint replacement. The role of stress analysis in the design of total joint replacements will, therefore, be illustrated by considering in detail one particular joint component, the femoral component of total hip replacements, with the hope that the reader will then be able to apply the same general principles to other types of prosthesis, a few of which will be dealt with briefly.

3.2 The Stems of the Femoral Components of Total Hip Replacements

A number of total hip replacement femoral stems have fractured while in use (see Chapter 1, section 2.3). One way of preventing future clinical fractures is to use stronger materials, and this possibility has been discussed in Chapter 1. A second way is to redesign the stems so as to reduce the stresses produced in them, and this is the approach discussed in the following sections.

3.2.1 THEORETICAL CONSIDERATIONS

Figure 2.10 is a schematic diagram of a cemented femoral component showing the resultant force (F) applied across the joint. The magnitude of this joint force varies during activity, and its direction and the position of the femur both vary in three-dimensional space. Other forces (not shown) acting on the structure include a frictional torque at the head and muscle forces at different points on the femur; these also vary in magnitude and direction with time. Together, the applied forces produce compressive stresses, bending stresses, shear stresses, and torsional stresses on every section, such as A–A, through the bone, cement and stem, and the magnitudes of these stresses vary from point to point across the section, and with time at each point.

Although the complete four-dimensional stress analysis of the structure is clearly impractical, simple stress analysis considerations can help to explain the occurrence of stem fracture and thereby suggest ways in which it might be avoided.

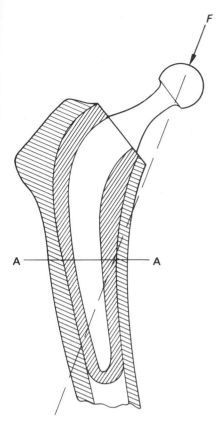

Figure 2.10.
A schematic diagram of a total hip replacement femoral component.

Metallurgical examination of removed fractured stems has shown that failure is caused by excessive tensile stress on the lateral surface (see Chapter 1, section 2.3). Tensile stresses in this region can only be produced by bending (i.e. with the head tending to move downwards and medially with respect to the stem). It follows that, since the magnitudes of the stresses produced by bending are inversely proportional to the flexural second moment of area of the cross-section and directly proportional to the bending moment (see section 1.2 of this chapter), there are two ways in which the stresses can be reduced. They are: (1) by increasing the flexural second moment of area of the stem cross-section; and (2) by reducing the magnitude of the bending moment. Since the force tending to bend the stem is the joint force (F), the bending moment about the stem can be reduced by reducing the moment arm of this force. This can be done by either reducing the curvature (or 'throw') of the stem itself and/or by increasing the inclination of the neck of the component to the horizontal. (Conversely, the varus positioning of a stem will increase the magnitude of the tensile stresses on the lateral surface by increasing the moment arm of the joint force.)

Recently a number of new femoral stem designs have been introduced which incorporate some or all of the above design changes (increased flexural second moment of area, reduced stem curvature, and increased neck inclination). Unfortunately, however, the situation is not as simple as it first appears and all of the changes have disadvantages which should be appreciated.

Firstly, as shown in section 1.6 of this chapter, the loads (compressive, bending, shear, and torsion) applied to composite structures are divided between the various elements of the structure in proportion to their relative stiffnesses (compressive stiffnesses, EA; flexural stiffnesses, EI_F; shear stiffnesses, GA; and torsional stiffnesses, GI_P). Thus, increasing the flexural second moment of area of a femoral stem increases the proportion of the applied bending moment carried by it. Although these two effects do not completely cancel and the magnitudes of the bending stresses in the stem are reduced, the effect on the cortical bone must be considered. In the normal femur the applied loads are carried entirely by the bone. Implanting a stem reduces the loads and therefore the stresses in the bone, and clearly the higher the proportion of the applied loads carried by the stem the lower will be the stresses in the bone. To the extent to which the turnover and remodelling of bone depends on mechanical stress (Wolff's law), this could be a serious problem since excessively stiff stems might well lead to disuse-osteoporosis.

Wilson and Scales (1970) have drawn attention to this problem. They state that disuse-atrophy of the calcar femorale and cervical stump can occur with a firmly cemented femoral component if the applied load is distributed to regions of bone distal to the transected neck. In the analysis of nine- and ten-year results with Charnley hips, Charnley and Cupic (1973) found some bone resorption in 44 of the 93 cases available for follow-up. Although they considered 3–4 mm resorption to be the 'normal' result of the interruption to the blood supply, 20 cases out of the 93 showed more than 4 mm and 3 showed more than 10 mm. It seems probable that in at least some of these cases resorption was the result of a decrease in mechanical loading (although other mechanisms, discussed in

Chapter 4, may also be at work). In a later paper, Charnley (1975) reviewed the cases of stem fracture in his prosthesis and concluded that lack of support to the proximal stem due to resorption of the calcar was one of the major factors contributing to fracture. This suggests something of a vicious circle—increasing the stiffness of a stem so as to reduce the stresses in it also reduces the stresses in the proximal bone; this leads to bone resorption, leaving the proximal stem unsupported and this is turn increases the stresses in the stem.

Secondly, decreasing the moment arm of the joint force about the stem, by reducing the curvature of the stem or by increasing the neck angle, or both, has two disadvantages. Firstly, by displacing the femur medially with respect to the pelvis the moment arm of the abductor muscles is reduced and this will increase the magnitude of the joint force. Although the net effect might be a reduction in the tensile stresses in the lateral surface of the stem, the increased load is likely to increase the rate of wear at the articulating surfaces (see Chapter 3). Secondly, reducing the bending moment by reducing the moment arm will reduce the stresses in the proximal bone as well as those in the stem, and this could lead to an increased incidence of osteoporosis.

Figure 2.11.
Details of the femoral components tested by Weightman (1976). (a) an original Charnley component, manufactured by Thackray Ltd. (b) a Charnley Extra-Heavy ('cobra') component, manufactured by Thackray Ltd. (c) a CAD Standard Curved (Vitallium[R] CAD[TM]) component, manufactured by Howmedica Ltd. (d) a CAD Standard Straight (Vitallium[R] CAD[TM]) component, manufactured by Howmedica Ltd. The figure shows the stem profiles, the cross-sections at mid-stem, and the position of the clamp in the distal fixation test.

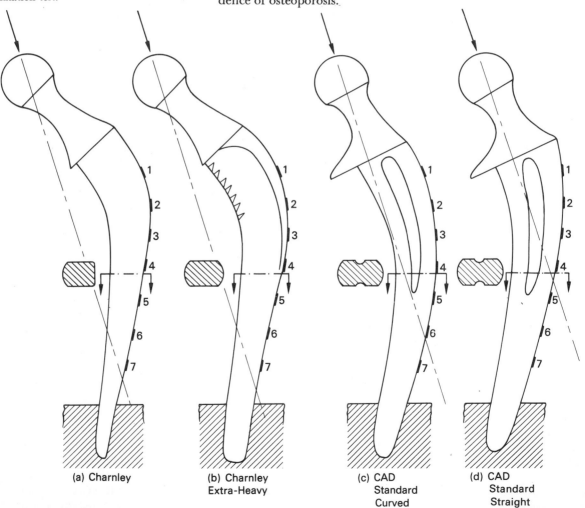

(a) Charnley

(b) Charnley Extra-Heavy

(c) CAD Standard Curved

(d) CAD Standard Straight

3.2.2 EXPERIMENTAL STRESS
ANALYSIS

A number of workers have measured the stresses produced in femoral stems in simplified laboratory tests. Markolf and Amstutz (1976) studied the effect of fixation breakdown by loading strain-gauged femoral components in three types of test: (1) with the stems securely fixed into blocks of cement; (2) with the stems loose in blocks of cement; and (3) with the stems fixed in blocks of cement by the distal third only. These tests showed that the tensile stresses in the lateral surface of the stems were much higher when they were loose or supported only distally than when rigidly fixed over their entire length. Other tests with the stems held at different angles in the medial-lateral plane showed that the stress levels were increased when the stems were in varus. Markolf and Amstutz concluded that inadequate proximal-medial support due to either poor quality bone or cement fracture, varus placement, and inadequate stem design could all contribute to dangerously high stress levels in femoral stems.

Weightman (1976) compared the stress levels in a number of different designs of femoral stem and it is interesting to compare the results with theoretical predictions.

Figure 2.11 shows the components tested, with strain gauges attached to the lateral surface of each stem. The seven gauge positions are indicated by the numbers 1–7, and are referred to by these numbers in Fig. 2.12. Two series of tests were conducted: (1) with the stems clamped at their tip as shown in Fig. 2.11; and (2) with the stems cemented over their entire length into post-mortem femora. In both series the problem was simplified to two dimensions by considering only one value of applied load and applying it in the plane of the stems. The load used was 4 kN (approximately six times the body weight of a heavy person) and it was applied at an angle of 14° to the vertical with the stems at an angle of 10° to the vertical, making a total angle of 24° between the load and stem axes.

Figure 2.12.
Stress profiles with the stems distally clamped. Graph of stress magnitude against strain gauge position. Applied load of 4 kN.

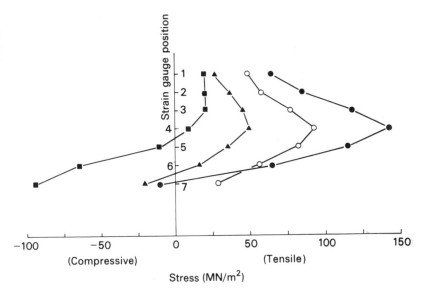

● Charnley
○ Charnley Extra-Heavy
▲ CAD Standard Curved
■ CAD Standard Straight

39

The comparative results were in close agreement with the theoretical predictions. That is, when the stems were clamped at their tips and loaded, maximum tensile stresses in the lateral surfaces (Fig. 2.12) decreased in the order Charnley, Charnley Extra-Heavy, CAD Standard Curved, and CAD Standard Straight, because, compared with the Charnley:

(1) the Charnley Extra-Heavy has a larger flexural second moment of area;

(2) the CAD Standard Curved has a larger flexural second moment of area, and an increased neck angle;

(3) the CAD Standard Straight has a larger flexural second moment of area, an increased neck angle and a reduced stem curvature.

Figure 2.13.
Stress profiles with stems cemented in bone. Graph of stress magnitude against strain gauge position. Applied load of 4 kN.

● Charnley

○ Charnley Extra-Heavy

▲ CAD Standard Curved

■ CAD Standard Straight

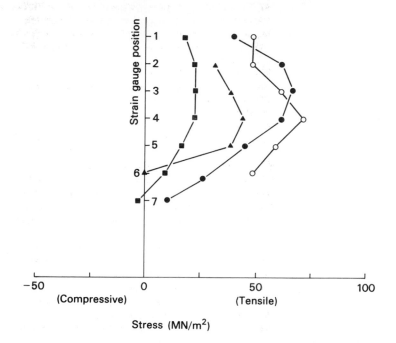

When the stems were cemented in post-mortem femora and reloaded (Fig. 2.13) (i.e. when a composite structure was formed and loaded in compression) the maximum tensile stress in the Charnley stem was reduced by approximately 50 per cent, presumably because a high proportion of the applied load was being carried by the bone instead of the stem. In the Charnley Extra-Heavy and the CAD Standard Curved, the maximum tensile stresses were reduced by 25 and 10 per cent respectively, indicating that for reasons set out in section 1.6.1 above, a smaller fraction of the applied load was being transferred to the proximal bone as the stiffness of the stems increased. (With the CAD Standard Straight the maximum tensile stress actually increased slightly, but this was thought to be due to the slight varus positioning of this prosthesis in the femur which increased the moment arm from one test to the other.)

More recent experimental work (Weightman, Abdulmihsein, Boiling and Wisnom, unpublished) seems to confirm that the insertion of a stiff femoral stem and an increasing neck angle both decrease the stresses in the proximal cortical bone. Strain gauges were attached to the medial and lateral surfaces of a post-mortem human femur at the positions shown in Fig. 2.14b and the femur was loaded, in the same direction as in the previous tests, through a soft rubber cap moulded to fit the superior surface of the head. A CAD Standard Curved femoral component was then inserted and the test repeated. Figures 2.14a and c show the resulting comparative stress profiles for the medial and lateral surfaces respectively.

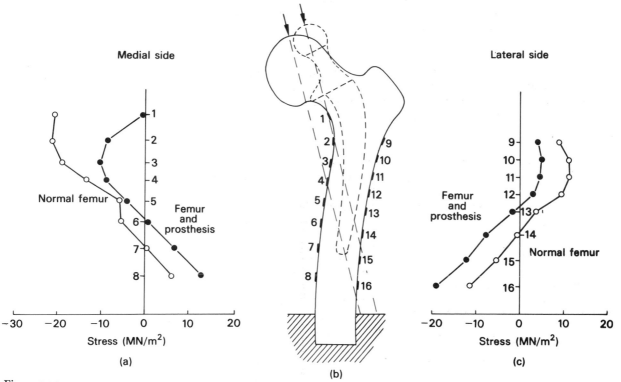

Figure 2.14.
The effect of a femoral stem on the stresses in the proximal femur. Graphs of stress magnitude against strain gauge position for a normal femur and a normal femur with a CAD Standard Curved femoral component cemented in. Applied load of 4 kN.

The greater inclination to the horizontal of the neck of the prosthesis compared with the natural neck had the effect of displacing the line of action of the applied load laterally when the prosthesis was inserted. This reduced the moment arm of the load about the proximal bone (anti-clockwise bending moment) but increased the moment arm about the distal bone (clockwise bending moment). Comparing the results for strain gauges 8 and 16, where the prosthetic stem itself should have little or no effect, it would appear that the displacement of the line of action of the applied load increases the tensile stress by approximately 8 MN/m² medially (Fig. 2.14a) and decreases the compressive stress by a similar amount laterally. If it is assumed that the displacement of the load line produces these effects over the entire length of the structure (i.e. produces stresses 8 MN/m² more tensile on the medial surface and 8 MN/m² more compressive on the lateral surface), then the results shown in Fig. 2.14c indicate that the greater neck angle of the prosthesis almost completely explains the differences in the two stress profiles on the lateral surface. However, the same argument cannot explain the much larger reduction in compressive stress in the proximal-medial bone (from approximately 21 MN/m^2 to 0·7 MN/m^2 under strain gauge 1, a factor of 30), and hence a large proportion of this reduction is apparently due to the effect of the stem itself.

It is interesting to note that the reduction in stress in the proximal-medial bone occurred even with the large neck collar of the CAD Standard Curved component. Clearly the collar was not fulfilling its intended purpose of transferring a relatively high proportion of the applied load directly to the proximal-medial cortical bone. Since there is no reason to suppose that the collars on any other type of femoral component would behave any differently, the results of this experiment therefore bring into question the usefulness of neck collars.

3.2.3 SUMMARY AND CONCLUSIONS

Both theoretical and experimental stress analysis lead to the following conclusions concerning the design of total hip replacement femoral components with intramedullary stems.

(1) When a femoral component stem is cemented into a femur a high proportion of the applied load is transmitted by the stem to the distal bone and so bypasses the proximal bone. The stresses in the proximal bone are therefore lower than in the normal femur and this may lead to disuse-osteoporosis and resorption of the calcar (see Chapter 5, section 2.2).

(2) Increasing the flexural second moment of area of the stem cross-section and decreasing the moment arm of the applied load about the proximal stem (by increasing the inclination of the neck and/or reducing the curvature of the stem) both reduce the magnitudes of the tensile stresses produced in the lateral surface of the stem, and therefore reduce the likelihood of stem fracture. However, each of these design changes further reduces the magnitude of the stresses in the proximal bone and hence increases the likelihood of disuse-osteoporosis.

(3) More work is required to establish the optimum design of femoral components which would minimise both stem fracture and disuse-osteoporosis.

3.3 Stress Analysis of Other Components

Few components have been investigated as thoroughly as the stems of the femoral components of hip prostheses, but in principle every section of every component should be examined to ensure that excessive stresses will not arise in service. In practice, manufacturing or other considerations mean that many sections of many components are of such dimensions that dangerously high stresses cannot arise, and it is thus only necessary to examine a few critical sections. The examination can be theoretical or experimental or both; experimental stress analysis will usually be resorted to only if the theoretical analysis suggests that dangerous stresses may arise but cannot be calculated with enough accuracy. A few examples follow.

The neck of the femoral component of a hip is loaded in a combination of compression, shear and bending (Fig. 2.15). If the neck is circular in cross-section, the stresses resulting from each of these components of load can be calculated by the methods referred to earlier in this chapter, if the magnitude and direction of the result-

Figure 2.15.
The neck of the femoral component of a hip prosthesis, showing (a) the resultant force applied to the femoral head, (b) this force replaced by components acting along and perpendicular to the axis of the neck, and balanced by a moment and two forces at the lateral end of the neck, (c) the shear stress at that section, (d) the compressive stress at that section, and (e) the bending stresses, varying from tension at the superior surface to compression at the inferior surface.

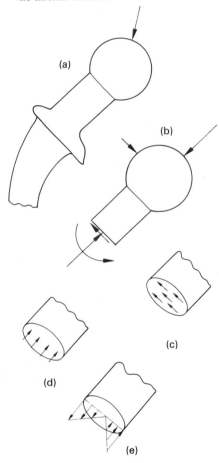

Figure 2.16.
A hinged knee prosthesis, showing (a) hyperextension resisted by an internal stop, (b) an adducting or abducting moment transmitted through the hinge, (c) the force system on the femoral component corresponding to (a), resulting in a bending moment in the stem, and (d) the force system in the tibial component corresponding to (b), resulting in a bending moment in the stem.

ant force on the femoral head are known. The limits on the knowledge of this force thus limit the accuracy with which the stresses can be predicted. Obviously, a thinner neck will experience higher stresses for a given load (the bending stresses vary inversely with the cube of the diameter of the cross-section, whereas the compressive and shear stresses vary inversely as its square); for a given direction of force on the femoral head, a more nearly horizontal neck will be subjected to a larger bending moment and hence higher bending stresses; a neck with its axis along the line of action of the resultant force on the femoral head would experience compressive stresses but neither bending nor shear stresses. This last condition could exist only at certain instants in a cycle of load and motion, but some designers have thought it worth arranging the geometry to reduce the bending and shear stresses at the instants when they are at their maximum values.

The stem of a hinged knee prosthesis is subjected to bending loads when motion is limited by a flexion or hyperextension stop, or when ab- or adducting moments are applied to the lower leg and resisted by the rest of the body (Fig. 2.16). The former bending loads act in the sagittal plane and the latter in the frontal, and the stem must therefore be designed to transmit all of them at safe levels of stress. An obvious difficulty arises, that the loads applied in these ways are not easy to predict, because they will normally arise dynamically rather than statically and may arise accidentally. Nevertheless, some attempt must be made to estimate them and to design the stems, particularly their junctions with the body of the prosthesis (where the stresses are likely to be greatest) to prevent fracture, on the basis that in the limit it is better for the prosthesis to loosen than for it to break.

Knee replacements of the resurfacing type often have femoral components of a generally U-shape as seen laterally. When loaded in flexion, as in stair-climbing, such a component can be compressed

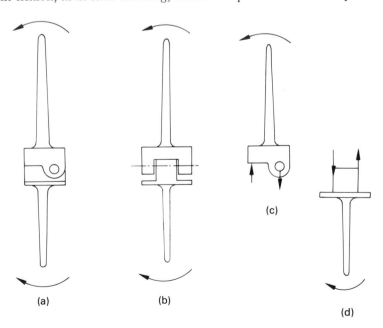

by forces applied by the tibial plateau and by forces applied through the patella, an intramedullary stem or spikes fixed by cement or otherwise in the cancellous bone of the femoral condyles.

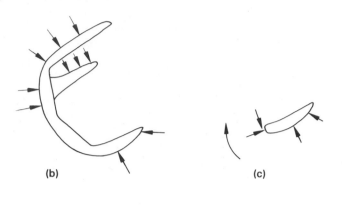

(b)

(c)

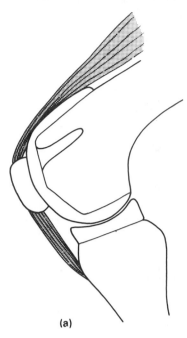

(a)

Figure 2.17.
(a) A representative surface replacement type of knee prosthesis in a position of about 80° of flexion. (b) A free body diagram of the femoral component, showing the forces exerted on it. If for any reason such as defective cementing the posterior portion is not supported by the posterior of the femoral condyles, the force system will be as shown and the femoral component will be subjected to a bending load, resisted by an internal bending moment as shown in (c).

Figure 2.18.
(a) The glenoid component of a shoulder prosthesis, consisting of a ball, a stalk and a base screwed to the bone. (b) A free body diagram of the stalk and ball, showing compressive force, shear force and bending moment in the stalk.

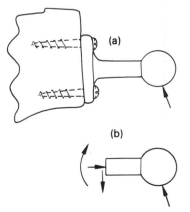

(a)

(b)

As shown in Fig. 2.17, these forces tend to bend the femoral component so as to increase its curvature. If the femoral component is attached to the femur in an ideal fashion, the forces will be transmitted to the bone of the femur and the femoral component of the prosthesis will experience local compression. If, however, the fixation is defective, some parts of the prosthetic component may be unsupported and then bending stresses will arise. Attempting to calculate these is very much a matter of engineering judgement: if the worst possible conditions are assumed, the prosthetic component may be unnecessarily heavy because it is stronger than it will ever need to be, but if no allowance is made for the possibility of partial fixation, an occasional fracture may occur.

Some shoulder replacement prostheses consist of a ball-and-socket joint, one component of which is attached to the glenoid area of the scapula by screws or other mechanical devices. Forces applied to the joint through the humerus will, in general, be transmitted to the glenoid anchorage partly as bending moments in the stalk joining the ball (or socket) to this anchorage, as shown in Fig. 2.18. As in the femoral neck, the corresponding bending stresses will be accompanied by shear stresses, but may be accompanied also by either tensile or compressive stresses if the joint is fully constrained. An acceptable range of movement is obtained more easily if the stalk is thin, but it must not be so thin that the stresses are too high. As in the femoral neck, the calculation of the bending, shear and tensile (or compressive) stresses presents no difficulty if the applied loads are known. At the shoulder, one could estimate the forces which could be transmitted through the humerus in various directions, but it would be almost impossible to estimate at all accurately the force arising when the elbow is accidentally struck, or even when the user leans on the elbow. One could instead measure in the laboratory the strength of the screws or other fixation arrangements in the glenoid area, and design the stalk to be safe at the loads corresponding to this strength, on the valid ground that loads higher than this applied to the joint will cause it to loosen from the scapula and any extra strength in the components would be redundant.

BIBLIOGRAPHY

Experimental Stress Analysis. (1965) J. W. Dally and W. F. Riley. New York and Maidenhead, McGraw-Hill.

Strength of Materials, Part İ, *Elementary Theory and Problems.* (1955) S. Timoshenko. New York and Wokingham, D. Van Nostrand.

REFERENCES

Charnley, J. (1975) Fracture of femoral prostheses in total hip replacement. A clinical study. *Clinical Orthopaedics and Related Research* **111,** 105.

Charnley, J. and Cupic, Z. (1973) The nine and ten year results of the low-friction arthroplasty of the hip. *Clinical Orthopaedics and Related Research* **95,** 9.

Markolf, K. L. and Amstutz, H. C. (1976) A comparative experimental study of stresses in femoral total hip replacement components: The effects of prosthesis orientation and acrylic fixation. *Journal of Biomechanics* **9,** 73.

Weightman, B. (1976) The stresses in total hip prosthesis femoral stems: a comparative study. In, International Symposium on Advances in Artificial Hip and Knee Joint Technology, Erlangen, W. Germany. *Engineering in Medicine*, Vol. 2. Berlin, Springer-Verlag. In the press.

Wilson, J. N. and Scales, J. T. (1970) Loosening of total hip replacements with cement fixation. Clinical findings and laboratory studies. *Clinical Orthopaedics and Related Research* **72,** 145.

CHAPTER THREE

Friction, Lubrication and Wear

MANY factors, both physiological and mechanical, affect the life of total joint replacement prostheses. One of these is wear of the joint components, since clinical and histopathological experience has shown that failure may result from gross wear (wearing out) or the tissue reaction to wear debris. In the first section of this chapter an attempt has been made to provide the basic engineering knowledge required for an understanding of the wear behaviour of materials. The second section reviews previous work on the wear of artificial joint materials in the light of this basic theory. Finally, examples are given of the way in which theory and clinical experience can combine to help the designer to produce improved total joint prostheses.

1 BASIC THEORY

Any discussion of the theory of wear must start with a consideration of friction.

Friction is the resistance to motion which exists between contacting solid bodies when an attempt is made to move one of the bodies tangentially relative to the other.

The origin of frictional forces can best be explained by reference to a simple model. On a microscopic scale all machined surfaces are rough, and two bodies in contact have been likened to Austria inverted and placed on Switzerland. Thus, when two bodies are pressed together under load (Fig. 3.1) contact takes place at surface asperities. Within the areas of real contact, atoms in the surface of one body are in intimate contact with atoms in the surface of the other body and the resulting interatomic forces produce adhesive junctions. Since these junctions must be broken before the two bodies can slide relative to each other, the force required to produce sliding, that is, the frictional force, is the force required to shear the junctions.

Although this is a considerably simplified model it explains why, in most cases, the frictional force between two bodies is directly proportional to load. In most metal-to-metal contacts the localised contact stresses exceed the hardness of the metal and plastic deformation takes place. The deformation continues until the area of real contact is sufficient to support the applied load. In the limit, the area of real contact increases until the contact stress is equal to the hardness of the metal. The total area of real contact is therefore given by

$$A_r = \frac{L}{p} \qquad \ldots (1)$$

where A_r is the real area of contact,
L is the applied load, and
p is the hardness.

The force necessary to shear the junctions (i.e. the frictional force) will be given by

$$F = A_r . s \qquad \ldots (2)$$

where s is the shear strength of the junctions.

Combining equations (1) and (2) gives

$$F = \frac{L.s}{p} \qquad \ldots (3)$$

Thus the frictional force is directly proportional to the load and the coefficient of friction, defined as the ratio of frictional force to load (F/L), is independent of load. These relationships can be considered the first 'law' of sliding friction. Two other 'laws', that the frictional force is independent of the area of contact and independent of sliding velocity, are also explained by the above analysis since equation (3) does not contain terms for either area of contact or sliding velocity.

Although the three laws are obeyed reasonably well in most cases,

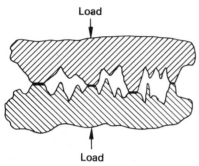

Load

Load

Figure 3.1.
Schematic diagram of two solid bodies in loaded contact.

there are exceptions. For example, with polymers the frictional force is not directly proportional to load and consequently the coefficient of friction varies with load. The reason for this behaviour is that polymer asperities can deform sufficiently to provide the required real area of contact without yielding. In this situation the real area of contact is not directly proportional to load. If the deformation is completely elastic, theory predicts that the real area of contact is proportional to load to the power 2/3. That is,

$$A_r = b.L^{0.67}$$

where b is a constant.

It follows from equation (2) that the frictional force is also proportional to load to this power, and that the coefficient of friction (F/L) is a function of load. In practice it is found that the frictional force on polymeric materials is proportional to load to a power between 0·67 (for purely elastic deformations) and 1·0 (for purely plastic deformations), and that the coefficient of friction decreases correspondingly with increasing load.

Experience has shown the third law (i.e. frictional force is independent of velocity) to be only approximately true. For instance, the force necessary to initiate sliding is greater than the force necessary to maintain sliding. This fact is normally accounted for by referring to the ratio of frictional force to load before sliding begins as the coefficient of static friction or the coefficient of stiction. Experiments have also shown that the coefficient of friction during sliding varies with sliding speed. With metals the coefficient of friction normally decreases with increasing speed, but in many cases so slowly that it can be considered to be a constant over practical ranges of velocity. With polymers, on the other hand, the coefficient of friction generally increases rapidly as the sliding speed increases and this is thought to be due to viscoelastic (time-dependent) properties of polymeric materials (see Chapter 1, section 1.1).

Since equation (3) does not include a term for the surface roughness of the sliding bodies, the model for friction predicts that this parameter has no effect on the frictional force. Although this is generally found to be the case over a wide range of surface finishes commonly used in engineering, very smooth and very rough surfaces can behave differently. Since the area of contact between two very smooth surfaces can be much greater than predicted in the above analysis, the force necessary to shear the junctions (i.e. the frictional force) can be much greater than expected. (If the two surfaces were 'perfectly' smooth and congruent, the real area of contact would equal the apparent area of contact at all loads.) With two very rough, hard surfaces the asperities tend to lock and an extra force must be applied in order to lift the asperities on the upper surface over those on the bottom surface. When a rough, hard surface slides over the surface of a softer material the hard asperities plough through the softer material and the frictional force is greater than would be expected on the basis of the shear strength of the junctions alone. In general then, the coefficient of friction between sliding bodies is independent of surface roughness over a wide range but can increase significantly for (1) two very smooth surfaces, (2) two very rough hard surfaces, and (3) a rough hard surface on a soft surface.

1.2 Types of Wear

Wear may be defined as the removal of material from solid surfaces during sliding. When the adhesive junctions formed between contacting solids are sheared during sliding, the shearing process may occur at different sites. If the interface at the junctions is weaker than either material, shearing will occur at the interface and only a very small amount of material will be removed from either surface. Since most interfaces are likely to contain imperfections this is probably the situation at most of the junctions formed between sliding materials. It follows that only a small proportion of the junctions formed between sliding bodies contribute to the wear process. If the interface is stronger than one material but weaker than the other, shearing will occur in the weaker (softer) material, leaving fragments adhering to the stronger (harder) surface. Thirdly, if the interface is stronger than one and occasionally stronger than the other, there will be marked transfer of the weaker material and some transfer of the stronger material. It has been found experimentally that even with materials of widely different hardness there is always some transfer of the harder material to the softer, presumably because there are local regions of low strength in hard materials and local regions of high strength in soft materials. Finally, if the interface is always stronger than both materials, shearing will take place away from the interface and heavy material transfer will occur. A good example of this is the case of identical metals in contact where the metal immediately to each side of the interface is strengthened by work-hardening, while that further away is not.

It is clear that the different events described above will produce widely differing wear rates, whereas the variation in frictional force will be far less. This explains why there is no clear relationship between wear rate and coefficient of friction.

The wear process which occurs when adhesively formed junctions shear elsewhere than at the interface is known as adhesive wear. A second type of wear, abrasive wear, occurs when either a rough surface ploughs through a softer material (two-body abrasive wear), or hard particles, trapped between the sliding surfaces, become attached to one surface and plough through the other (three-body abrasive wear). Although two-body abrasive wear can be avoided relatively easily by making the surface of the hard material smooth, three-body abrasive wear often results from particles produced by adhesive wear and is thus more difficult to prevent.

Other forms of wear include corrosive wear, surface fatigue wear, and brittle fracture wear. Corrosive wear occurs when materials slide against each other in a corrosive environment. In cases where the products of corrosion would not normally protect the material from further corrosion their removal by wear has little effect, and the rate of loss of material is essentially independent of sliding. In cases where the corrosion products do form protective layers the rate of loss of material depends on the wear resistance of these layers. If the layer is easily worn away, active corrosion of the base material will ensue. If, on the other hand, the protective film has a greater wear resistance than the parent material the corrosive environment will actually reduce the rate of material loss.

Corrosion is an electrochemical process (see Chapter 1, section 1.5) and can therefore only occur in metallic materials. However, polymers and ceramics can react chemically with their environment and this can produce a decrease in their mechanical properties, including wear resistance. Thus degradative wear of polymers and ceramics may be thought of as analogous to corrosive wear of metals.

In many situations, for example in ball bearings, surfaces experience repetitive contact. The continual loading and unloading which this produces can lead to surface fatigue wear. After a time (number of cycles), which depends on the magnitude of the load, surface or subsurface cracks are produced and, as these spread, relatively large fragments become detached from the surface. The site of the initial cracks, either surface or subsurface, depends on the relative strengths of a particular material in tension and shear. As an area of loaded contact moves over a surface, a complex pattern of stress is produced beneath the junction. The maximum shear stress is produced some distance below the contact surface whereas the maximum tensile stress is produced at the surface immediately behind the junction. Ductile materials fail by a shear mechanism (see Chapter 1, section 1.1) and therefore fatigue wear in ductile materials is likely to be initiated by subsurface cracks. Brittle materials, on the other hand, have low tensile strengths and are likely to fracture on the surface.

In extremely brittle materials the tensile stress behind a sliding junction may be sufficient to cause fracture of the surface on one pass. The resulting detachment of particles from the surface is known as brittle fracture wear, and Fig. 3.2 shows the characteristic appearance of wear tracks resulting from this type of wear.

The various combinations of materials used for total joint replacements are discussed in the light of these considerations in section 2 of this chapter.

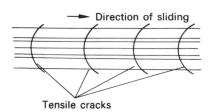

Figure 3.2.
The characteristic appearance of brittle fracture wear (Rabinowicz 1966).

1.3 The Laws of Wear

1.3.1 ADHESIVE WEAR

In general, the volume of debris produced by adhesive wear is found to be proportional to the load across the contacting surfaces and the sliding distance, and inversely proportional to the hardness of the surface being worn. That is, in most cases adhesive wear obeys the equation

$$v = \frac{c.L.x}{p} \qquad \ldots (4)$$

where c is a constant (called the coefficient of wear),
L is the load,
x is the distance traversed, and
p is the hardness of the surface being worn.

The equation can be explained in terms of a simple model. If d is the effective diameter of the junctions, the total real area of contact is given by

$$A_r = n.\frac{\pi d^2}{4} \qquad \ldots (5)$$

where n is the number of junctions.

By the time the two materials have moved a distance d, the junctions have sheared. If the proportion of junctions which produce a wear fragment is k, and the shape of each fragment is hemispherical, then the volume of wear produced in sliding a distance d is given by

$$v_d = k.n.\frac{\pi d^3}{12}$$

The volume of wear produced in sliding any distance x is therefore given by

$$v = k.n.\frac{\pi d^3}{12}.\frac{x}{d} = k.n.\frac{\pi d^2}{12}.x$$

But

$$n.\frac{\pi d^2}{4} = A_r$$

from equation (5) and

$$A_r = \frac{L}{p}$$

from equation (1), therefore

$$v = \frac{k}{3}.\frac{L}{p}.x$$

This adhesive wear equation based on a simple model is exactly the same as the experimentally derived equation (4), except that the constant c has been replaced by $k/3$.

1.3.2 ABRASIVE WEAR

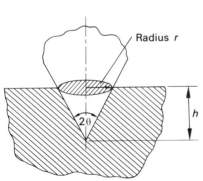

Figure 3.3.
Conical asperity for abrasive wear model.

The volume of wear produced by a hard asperity ploughing through a soft material is given by the product of the projected cross-sectional area of the asperity below the surface of the soft material and the distance travelled. A simple model for abrasive wear can be obtained if the asperities are assumed to be conical. Figure 3.3 shows such an asperity with a cone angle of 2θ. The volume of wear produced when this asperity ploughs a distance x through the soft material is given by

$$v = r.h.x$$

where h is the depth of penetration of the asperity.
But, since

$$\frac{r}{h} = \tan \theta,$$

$$v = \frac{r^2.x}{\tan \theta}$$

The projected area of contact (A_r) is given by

$$A_r = \pi r^2 = \frac{L}{p}$$

from equation (1); therefore

$$v = \frac{L}{p} \cdot \frac{x}{\pi \tan \theta}$$

This equation is similar to the adhesive wear equation (equation 4) in that the volume of wear is directly proportional to the load and the sliding distance, and inversely proportional to the hardness of the softer material. The only difference between the two wear equations is that the constant c in equation (4) is replaced by $1/\pi \tan \theta$. Tan θ is a shape factor related to the roughness of the abrasive surface. It can be seen that when $\theta = 90°$ the cone becomes a flat surface, tan θ equals infinity, and the equation predicts zero volume of abrasive wear.

1.3.3 THE 'P.V' RELATIONSHIP

In industry the wear resistances of different materials for use in dry and boundary-lubricated bearings are often compared on the basis of their limiting $P.V$ values (pressure × sliding velocity) as given by the manufacturers. Experience has shown that the rate of depth wear in dry and boundary-lubricated bearings is proportional to the product of nominal pressure (load divided by projected area of contact) and sliding velocity, and therefore a certain 'acceptable' rate of depth wear (arbitrarily fixed) is associated with a constant $P.V$ value. In practice it is extremely difficult to compare the $P.V$ values given by different manufacturers for different materials because the conditions under which they were obtained vary and are not usually stated.

The wear relationship on which the use of $P.V$ values is based is

$$h_t = k.P.V \qquad \qquad \dots (6)$$

where h_t is the rate of depth wear,
  P is the nominal contact pressure,
  V is the sliding velocity, and
  k is a constant.

It can be shown that this equation is merely the basic wear equation

$$v = \frac{c.L.x}{p}$$

in a different form. Thus, in a certain time (t) the depth wear (h) is given by

$$h = k.P.V.t$$

Since velocity multiplied by time $(V.t)$ equals sliding distance (x),

$$h = k.P.x$$

Since P equals load (L) divided by projected area of contact (A)

$$h.A = k.L.x$$

Since $h.A$ is equal to the volume of wear,

$$v = k.L.x$$

This equation is the basic wear equation (4), with the constant c/p replaced with the constant k.

1.4 Lubrication

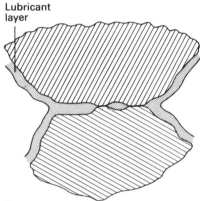

Lubricant layer

Figure 3.4.
Schematic diagram of a boundary lubricated junction.

Lubrication may be defined as the reduction produced in the inter-action between two contacting solid bodies by the introduction of a substance between them.

There are two main types of lubrication: fluid lubrication and boundary lubrication. In fluid lubrication the surfaces in relative motion are separated by a lubricant layer of appreciable thickness. Under ideal conditions the two solids are completely separated and there is no wear. The characteristics of fluid lubrication depend on the properties of the lubricant, the resistance to motion, for example, being controlled by the viscosity of the fluid layer. One of the most important types of fluid lubrication, hydrodynamic lubrica-tion, is produced when the pressure developed in a converging film of liquid between two solids is sufficient to keep the two surfaces apart. A good example is a journal bearing where a shaft rotating at high speed forces lubricant into a converging wedge produced by the displacement of the centre of the shaft from the centre of the bearing. Unfortunately, in other situations it is often impossible to produce hydrodynamic lubrication, especially if sliding speeds are low and/or loads are high.

In boundary lubrication the solid surfaces are separated by an extremely thin lubricant layer of only molecular dimensions. The fact that boundary lubrication does not completely eliminate wear indicates that the solid surfaces are not completely separated. It appears that boundary lubrication reduces but does not eliminate the area of contact of two surfaces at asperities. This situation is shown schematically in Fig. 3.4. Clearly, the resistance to sliding consists partly of the force necessary to shear the 'microjunctions' between the two surfaces and partly the force necessary to shear the lubricant itself. As well as explaining the fact that wear occurs when two solids are boundary lubricated, this model is consistent with the observations that the characteristics of boundary lubrication depend on the nature of the solid surfaces, the chemical composition of the lubricant, and the extent to which the lubricant is adsorbed on the surfaces.

If A is the area which supports load, a is the fraction of this area over which the two solid surfaces are in contact, S_m is the shear strength of these 'microjunctions', and S_1 is the shear strength of the boundary lubricant film, equation (2) (section 1.1) for materials in unlubricated contact can be adapted to give

$$F = a.A.S_m + (1-a)A.S_1$$

Since with most boundary lubricants a is small, the 'micro-junctions' contribute little to the frictional resistance. They are, however, responsible for wear, and this explains why different boundary lubricants can give dramatically different wear rates with similar coefficients of friction.

Other types of lubrication include elastohydrodynamic and squeeze film lubrication. Elastohydrodynamic lubrication is a parti-cular type of hydrodynamic lubrication which occurs when the pressure generated in the lubricant film is sufficient to produce sig-nificant elastic deformation of the bearing surfaces.

When a bearing is loaded and the two surfaces approach one another it takes a finite time to squeeze out the lubricant. Squeeze film lubrication occurs if the load is applied intermittently for times short enough to squeeze out only some of the lubricant and if the film can be replenished when the load is removed.

1.5 Summary

1.5.1 FRICTION

In most cases the frictional force between two materials in unlubricated sliding contact is directly proportional to the load and is independent of the apparent area of contact, the sliding velocity, and the surface finishes. Important exceptions to these general rules include the increased frictional forces between (1) two extremely smooth surfaces, (2) two extremely rough, hard surfaces, and (3) a rough, hard surface on a soft surface.

1.5.2 WEAR

(1) The most commonly occurring types of wear in general engineering are adhesive wear and abrasive wear. Adhesive wear is produced when the junctions formed between contacting materials shear away from the interface. Abrasive wear is produced by the ploughing of a hard material through a softer material.

  In any given situation the relative importance of these two wear mechanisms depends largely on the surface finishes and the hardness of the contacting materials. For example, two smooth surfaces are likely to wear (initially at least) by an adhesive mechanism, whereas a soft material will wear by abrasion if a rough hard surface slides over it.

(2) Adhesive wear often leads to abrasive wear.

(3) With both adhesive and abrasive wear the volume of wear debris produced in a given time is, in many cases, found to be proportional to the load and the sliding distance, and inversely proportional to the hardness of the material being worn away.

(4) Other forms of wear include fatigue wear and brittle fracture wear. While these types of wear occur less frequently in general engineering than adhesive and abrasive wear, they can be more damaging since they can produce extremely high rates of wear.

(5) The presence of a corrosive environment may have a drastic effect on wear rate.

1.5.3 LUBRICATION

(1) Fluid lubrication completely separates the two sliding bodies so that the resistance to motion depends on the properties of the lubricant and there is virtually no wear.

(2) Boundary lubrication only partially separates the sliding bodies. Both the frictional force and the wear rate are reduced but wear is not eliminated. The effect of boundary lubrication is to reduce the frictional force by reducing the tangential stress necessary to shear the junctions between the two materials (s in equation 3), and to reduce the wear rate by reducing the coefficient of wear (c in equation 4).

  Readers wishing to extend their study of the basic theories and phenomena of friction, lubrication and wear are referred to the bibliography at the end of this chapter.

2 THE WEAR OF TOTAL JOINT REPLACEMENTS

A considerable amount of laboratory work has been carried out in order to study the friction, lubrication, and wear of artificial human joints. This work can be divided into three categories: (1) studies using relatively simple apparatus such as pin-on-disc machines, making little or no effort to reproduce physiological conditions; (2) work with joint simulators under approximately physiological conditions of motion and loading; and (3) the analysis by materials science techniques of joint prostheses removed from patients.

In addition to laboratory studies, clinical trials and long-term follow-up studies have provided a limited amount of direct data on the wear performance of implant materials *in vivo*.

In general terms, the work with machines of simple configuration has sought to provide rapid testing procedures to be used as initial screening tests for candidate materials; joint simulators have been used to provide more accurate tests of promising materials and to compare various types of existing prostheses under controlled laboratory conditions; and removed prostheses have been examined in order to study the wear mechanisms operating in prostheses under actual working conditions.

2.1 Screening Tests with Simple Machines

Figure 3.5.
Simple wear machines.

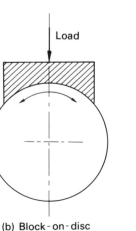

(a) Pin-on-disc

(b) Block-on-disc

A variety of machines using specimens of simple geometry have been used to study the wear of total joint replacement materials. They include:

(1) pin-on-disc machines (Fig. 3.5a), in which a pin is loaded against the flat surface of a rotating disc;
(2) block-on-disc machines (Fig. 3.5b), in which a loaded block conforms to the curved surface of an oscillating disc;
(3) disc-on-disc machines (Fig. 3.5c), in which a disc rotates with its curved surface loaded against the flat surface of a stationary disc;
(4) annulus-on-disc machines (Fig. 3.5d), in which an oscillating annulus is loaded with its flat surface against the flat surface of a stationary disc.

Tests with such machines have been run at different contact stresses and at different sliding speeds. Before describing some of the more important work it is therefore necessary to establish the approximate conditions under which total joint replacements operate *in vivo*.

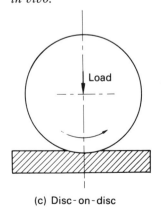

(c) Disc-on-disc

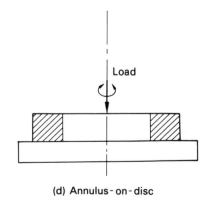

(d) Annulus-on-disc

The loads across hip joints fluctuate between approximately zero and some peak value during activity. While peak loads of six times body weight have been recorded during walking with some subjects, typical values are closer to four times body weight (Paul 1967). Artificial hip joints in vigorous patients having a body mass of 60 kg are therefore likely to experience peak loads of approximately 2·4 kN. The contact stresses produced in an artificial joint by a given load will vary over the area of contact in a way which depends on the geometry and mechanical properties of the two joint components. However, a first order approximation can be obtained by dividing the load by the projected area of contact (i.e. $\pi d^2/4$, where d is the diameter of the femoral head). This calculation yields values of peak nominal contact stress of approximately 6·3 MN/m² and 2·5 MN/m² for femoral heads of 22 mm and 35 mm diameter respectively.

Sliding speeds also vary between zero (at full extension and flexion) and some maximum. Paul (1967) estimated the highest sliding speed in the natural hip joint during normal walking to be about 0·08 m/s, while Charnley (1976) calculated the average sliding speed inside a prosthesis with a 20 mm diameter femoral head to be 0·012 m/s at a walking speed of 3·2 km/h (2 miles/h).

Conditions at joints other than the hip will vary more widely, and less is known about them; but the above gives an indication of the contract stresses and rubbing speeds which are likely to be relevant.

2.1.1 REVIEW OF THE LITERATURE

Walker et al. (1967) used a pin-on-disc machine to measure the friction and wear of artificial joint materials. Flat-ended cylindrical specimens were loaded, under a nominal contact pressure of 19·6 MN/m², against the flat surface of a rotating stainless steel disc. The sliding speed was 0·025 m/s and tests were run dry and with synovial fluid as lubricant. Wear of the pins was measured by weighing before and after five-hour tests. Materials tested included Perspex (polymethylmethacrylate), acetal copolymer, Nylon 66, high density polyethylene (a common term for the grade which is also of high molecular weight), polytetrafluorethylene (PTFE or Teflon), neoprene rubber and cellular polyurethane. The authors concluded that, within the limitations of the experiment, high density polyethylene was the best plastic for metal-to-plastic artificial joints.

Amstutz (1968) measured the friction and wear of ten different polymers when conforming blocks were loaded against the curved surface of an oscillating hardened steel ring. The oscillating frequency was 89 cycles per minute through a 90° arc (maximum sliding speed of 0·11 m/s), and the nominal contact stress (load divided by projected area) was 6·4 MN/m². After friction tests with a variety of lubricants, mineral oil was selected for the wear tests because it gave a similar coefficient of friction to synovial fluid. Wear rates were calculated from both dimensional changes and weight changes, but certain difficulties were encountered; creep, particularly of Delrin (polyacetal) and ultra-high molecular weight (uhmw) polyethylene, made dimensional changes difficult to measure; one specimen of uhmw polyethylene increased in weight due to mineral oil absorption before presoaking was introduced, and large variations in the wear rate of the same material were found in different series of identical tests (particularly with polyimide, Delrin, and polycarbonate). However, certain conclusions were reached, namely that polyimides and uhmw polyethylene exhibited the highest wear resistance while uhmw polyethylene and Delrin gave the lowest coefficients of friction.

Scales (1972) reported on the use of a pin-on-disc machine to study the wear of cobalt–chromium alloy, high density polyethylene and polyester discs when loaded against cobalt–chromium alloy pins with bovine serum as lubricant. The results showed that the volumetric wear of high density polyethylene was approximately 20 times that produced by the metal-on-metal combination. Of particular interest was the finding that, while autoclaved polyester had a lower wear rate than high density polyethylene, hydrolysis, which could occur in the body, had disastrous effects on its wear resistance.

Galante and Rostoker (1973) evaluated the wear of over 25 different materials and combinations of materials with a disc-on-disc specimen configuration (the curved surface of a rotating disc was loaded against the flat surface of a stationary disc). Two sliding speeds, 0·106 m/s and 1·483 m/s, were used; the nominal contact stress ranged from 2·1 to 6·9 MN/m²; and water at 37°C was used as lubricant in most of the tests.

Wear rates were obtained by dividing the depth of wear by the total sliding distance. Since the contact area increased during each test under a fixed load, each wear rate corresponded to a certain range of nominal contact stress. As Galante and Rostoker point out, if the basic wear equation

$$v_x = k'.L \quad \text{(see section 1.3, equation 4)}$$

where v_x is the volume of wear per unit sliding distance,
$\quad$ L is the load, and
$\quad$ k' is a constant equal to c/p,
is divided by the area of contact, it becomes

$$h_x = k'.P$$

where P is the nominal contact stress, and
$\quad$ h_x is the depth of wear per unit sliding distance.

This equation indicates a linear relationship between depth of wear per unit sliding distance and nominal contact stress. With most of the material combinations tested, Galante and Rostoker's experimental data did not support this relationship. Within the range of nominal contact stress considered relevant to total hip prostheses (approximately 2·0 MN/m² for a 35 mm diameter head to 5·5 MN/m² for a 22 mm diameter head) most of the materials tested showed depth wear rates increasing more rapidly than predicted. Galante and Rostoker suggested that this signified a gradual transition from a mild to a severe wear mechanism (i.e. changes in the wear factor k'), with increasing nominal contact stress, and emphasised the importance of this finding in the choice of femoral head diameter.

Ultra-high molecular weight polyethylene, however, was something of an exception. This material showed a region between 2·1 and 5·0 MN/m² in which its wear rate against Vitallium cast cobalt–chromium alloy was almost constant. Within the limits of experimental accuracy, it would appear that the wear of uhmw polyethylene agrees with theoretical predictions, although Galante and Rostoker did not comment on this point. Above 5 MN/m² the wear rate increased rapidly. When the reduction in sliding distance which accompanies a reduction in femoral head size was taken into account, Galante and Rostoker found that the ideal size of femoral head for use with uhmw polyethylene sockets is between 22 and 28 mm. (For a more detailed analysis of the factors affecting the choice of femoral head size, see section 3 of this chapter.)

Other conclusions were that: (1) uhmw polyethylene against Vitallium produced the lowest wear rates of the commercially available materials (i.e. lower than with either stainless steel or Ti–6Al–4V alloy); (2) the wear rates of ceramics such as aluminium oxide, silicon carbide and boron carbide against themselves were too high for total joint replacement use; and (3) at a nominal contact stress of 2·1 MN/m², a material consisting of uhmw polyethylene plus 25 per cent graphite powder had a wear rate between one-seventh and one-thirtieth that of uhmw polyethylene alone, but at higher nominal contact stresses the wear rate of the graphite-filled polyethylene approached that of the unfilled material.

Ungethüm and Refior (1974) used 6 mm diameter pins with spherical ends of 20 mm radius against rotating discs. The sliding speed was 0·05 m/s, the load was 100 N (contact pressure of 3·5 MN/m² at full contact), and tests were run for 48 hours either dry or with Ringer's solution as lubricant. The depth of the wear track on the discs was used as a measure of wear. Material combinations tested were cobalt–chromium alloy pins against polyester (Sulzer, AP4), cobalt–chromium alloy pins against high density polyethylene, aluminium oxide ceramic from three different German manufacturers against discs of the same material, and cobalt–chromium alloy against itself. After 48 hours the depths of the wear tracks on the discs were 15·7 μm for the polyester, 1·90 μm for the polyethylene, and 0·375, 0·438 and 0·950 μm for the three different Al₂O₃ ceramics. There was no measurable wear on the cobalt–chromium alloy disc. Although the Al₂O₃ combination appears at first sight to have a wear rate less than half that of polyethylene, the wear of the pins must be taken into account. In the case of cobalt–chromium pins against polyethylene this is probably negligible but with an Al₂O₃ pin against an Al₂O₃ disc wear of the pin is likely to be significant. (In a personal communication (1976) Ungethüm reports that the wear of the ceramic pins was 30 μm, 30 μm and 56 μm, respectively, but without more information it is still impossible to compare the different materials on the basis of volume of wear debris produced.)

Coefficients of friction in Ringer's solution were 0·26 to 0·35 for the ceramic combinations, 0·03 to 0·05 for polyethylene and polyester against cobalt–chromium alloy, and 0·3 to 0·4 for cobalt–chromium alloy on itself.

Since these workers were particularly interested in the use of ceramics in joint replacements, they examined the wear grooves on the aluminium oxide discs in a scanning electron microscope. They found holes produced by the tearing out of crystallites, wear tracks indicative of microscopic plastic deformation, and cracks thought to have been produced by fatigue.

Miller et al. (1974) used the flat surface of an oscillating metal annulus loaded against the flat surface of a stationary uhmw polyethylene specimen to compare the wear of the polymer when used in combination with cast cobalt–chromium alloy, stainless steel and Ti–6Al–4V alloy. Ringer's solution was used as lubricant, the average sliding speed was 0·018 m/s and a constant load gave a nominal contact pressure of 3·45 MN/m². Under these conditions the wear of the polyethylene (measured as depth wear after 5 km of sliding) was essentially the same with all three alloys.

Since the finding of Miller et al., that the wear of uhmw polyethylene is no greater when used with Ti–6Al–4V alloy than when used with cast cobalt–chromium alloy, conflicted with the earlier findings of Galante and Rostoker, these authors repeated their work (Rostoker and Galante, 1976). Using the same disc-on-disc machine, 16 individual tests were conducted. The contact pressures varied between 0·14 and 6·9 MN/m², tests were run dry and with water as lubricant, and various sliding velocities were used. Of the 16 tests, 12 developed an abnormally high wear rate within minutes to hours. Only 2 tests ran for a week (end of the test) with a relatively low wear rate. Rostoker and Galante concluded that the titanium alloy is unsuitable for use in combination with uhmw polyethylene.

2.1.2 DISCUSSION

Friction and wear tests with simple machines have a number of advantages and disadvantages. Apart from the simple geometry of the test specimens, other advantages include the relative ease with which wear can be measured and the fact that high speed rotation (or oscillation) can produce an accelerated wear test. Unfortunately, the type of lubrication produced between the sliding components (for example, boundary or hydrodynamic) depends to a large extent on the sliding speed, and the type of lubrication can have an enormous effect on wear rate. Laboratory studies with joint simulators (see section 2.2 of this chapter) have shown that total joint replacements are boundary lubricated. Thus, if hydrodynamic lubrication is produced in high speed wear tests, the wear results are unlikely to be relevant to the *in vivo* wear of total joint replacements. It also follows that if the conditions of the simple test are such as to produce boundary lubrication, the lubricant used is of major importance in determining the wear rates (see section 1.4 of this chapter).

Another criticism of these simplified tests concerns the effect of specimen geometry and the type of loading produced on the measured wear rates of polymers in polymer-on-metal combinations. In a pin-on-disc machine, for example, if a polymer pin and a metal disc are used, the pin is sliding under a constant load and possible fatigue wear (which might occur in the body as a result of the fluctuating loads across the joint) goes undetected. On the other hand, if a metal pin and a polymer disc are used, experience shows that an unrealistically high wear rate is produced. There appear to be two separate factors involved in this. Firstly, the metal pin indents into the polymer disc and hence tends to plough through it as the disc rotates (Fig. 3.6a). Secondly, although the polymer experiences a fluctuating load, the rate of loading, from the unloaded state immediately ahead of the pin to the fully loaded state under the pin, is extremely high. Polymers being viscoelastic materials have time-dependent mechanical properties (see Chapter 1, section 1.1), so that these high loading rates may well produce more damage than the almost certainly lower loading rates experienced *in vivo*.

Figure 3.6.
The effect of specimen configuration in simple wear machines. (X indicates regions of ploughing and high rates of loading).

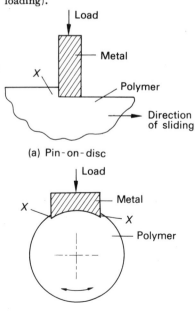

(a) Pin-on-disc

(b) Block-on-disc

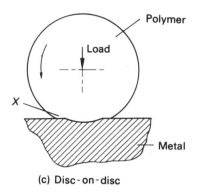

(c) Disc-on-disc

Figure 3.6 *cont.*

The same effects occur in block-on-disc and disc-on-disc machines; if the convex component (the rotating or oscillating disc) is polymeric, ploughing and high loading rates can combine to produce excessive wear (Fig. 3.6b and c). For this reason most investigators make the pins in pin-on-disc machines and the concave components in block-on-disc and disc-on-disc machines out of the polymeric material to be tested, and accept the criticism that the polymer is not experiencing fluctuating loads.

Although the problem of which component should be metal and which should be polymer has been discussed above as a criticism of wear tests of simple geometry, it is also important in the design of total joint replacements. In the most commonly used metal-on-polymer total hip and total knee replacements (for example, the Charnley and Charnley–Müller total hips and the Geomedic, Polycentric and ICLH total knees) the convex component is metallic and the concave component is polymeric. However, in a number of designs, including the Tronzo and Weber (polyester version) total hips and the Charnley total knee, the materials have been reversed (Fig. 3.7).

Figure 3.7.
Schematic diagram of total joint replacements with convex polymer components.

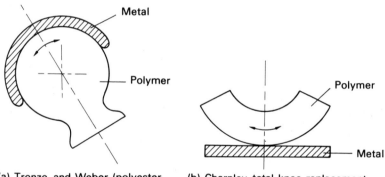

(a) Tronzo and Weber (polyester version) total hip replacements

(b) Charnley total knee replacement

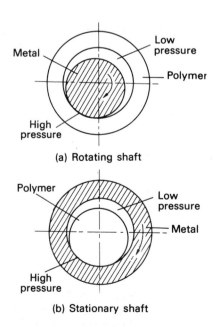

(a) Rotating shaft

(b) Stationary shaft

Figure 3.8.
Industrial metal-on-polymer bearings.

Although the ploughing effect of the metal edge is not present in these designs the polymer experiences high rates of loading in those areas which oscillate between loaded and unloaded positions. In laboratory wear tests during the development of the ICLH total hip joint and the ICLH total ankle joint, considerably more wear was observed when the convex component was polymer and the concave component was metal than vice versa (Day, Swanson and Freeman, unpublished data; and Kempson, Freeman and Tuke 1975). In industrial metal-on-polymer bearings the rotating component is always metal and the stationary component is always polymer, since this arrangement protects the polymer from rapidly changing loads (Fig. 3.8). It should be noted that the important consideration is not which component is concave and which convex, but which component experiences rapidly changing loads and which does not. Expressed another way, it is engineering practice to ensure that the 'metal surface always extends beyond the polymer bearing surface'. (This rule applies to the bearings shown in Fig. 3.8 since in (a) only part of the polymer bush is carrying load, and in (b) only part of the polymer shaft is carrying load.)

Thus theoretical considerations, laboratory experiments, and engineering experience all point to the fact that the decision on which components should be made out of which material in total joint replacements is a crucial one. It is important to ensure that the metal bearing surface extends beyond the polymer bearing surface, and in practice this means that the polymer component of total joint replacements should have a concave surface and the metallic component a convex surface.

2.1.3 SUMMARY

Although only a brief description of some of the work done with machines of simple geometry has been given above, and the relevance of this type of test to the *in vivo* situation can be questioned, the important results may be summarised as follows.

(1) Of the possible metal–metal combinations for use in total joint replacements, only cast cobalt–chromium alloy against itself is suitable.

(2) On the basis of wear rate and coefficient of friction, uhmw polyethylene is a better material for use in a polymer-on-metal joint than PTFE, polyacetal, polyester or Nylon.

(3) Ceramics such as aluminium oxide, silicon carbide and boron carbide appear to give high rates of wear and high coefficients of friction when sliding against themselves.

(4) The data on the use of Ti–6Al–4V against uhmw polyethylene are in conflict.

(5) In metal-on-polymer total joint replacements the concave component should be polymeric and the convex component metallic.

2.2 Laboratory Studies with Joint Simulators

2.2.1 REVIEW OF THE LITERATURE

A number of research groups have used joint simulators of varying degrees of sophistication to study the wear performance of total joint replacements.

Duff-Barclay and Spillman (1967) described results obtained from a hip joint simulator which closely reproduced the flexion–extension, adduction–abduction and internal–external rotation motions of the human hip and incorporated a fluctuating load cycle with a maximum load of approximately 1 kN. The running speed was 27 cycles per minute and tests of up to 200 hours duration were conducted under dry conditions and with saline and plasma as lubricants.

Of the metal–metal combinations tested only cast cobalt–chromium alloy against itself gave satisfactory results. The frictional effort required to articulate this combination was lower with plasma than with saline and this was attributed to the protein content of the plasma. The frictional characteristics with both lubricants were consistent with boundary lubrication.

A combination of cobalt–chromium alloy against high density polyethylene with plasma as lubricant was found to give low friction. Although there was no measurable wear after 200 hours the polyethylene cup was considerably distorted due to flow of the plastic. By contrast, a 500-hour test of a Charnley prosthesis showed significant polyethylene wear, apparently due to a fatigue mechanism, but no distortion. One possible explanation of these conflicting results was thought to be the more rigid support given to the Charnley cup; this may have prevented distortion and hence promoted fatigue wear.

A polyacetal (Delrin) acetabular cup was also found to wear by a fatigue mechanism when run with a cobalt–chromium femoral component.

These authors concluded that, of the materials tested, cast cobalt–chromium alloy against itself was the best for use in total joint replacements.

Using the same hip joint simulator but with the load cycle adapted to include a swing phase under zero load, Scales, Kelly and Goddard (1969) made a study of the frictional torque produced by total hip replacements. Using reconstituted human plasma as lubricant, frictional measurements were taken at intervals during 500-hour tests.

Metal-on-metal prostheses (cast cobalt–chromium alloy) exhibited a varying frictional resistance which was thought to be due to a running-in process. The importance of the design of the bearing, to ensure that contact occurred towards the apex (pole) of the cup, and of surface finish, in reducing frictional torque was emphasised. The authors considered that, since large frictional torques produce large stresses at the cup–cement and cement–bone interfaces, large torques could be the cause of prosthetic loosening in some cases.

Stainless steel and cobalt–chromium alloy were tested against high density polyethylene and both combinations were found to have less frictional resistance than metal-on-metal prostheses.

Walker and Gold (1971) measured the frictional torques generated when 10 McKee–Farrar prostheses, which had been removed from patients between 3 and 18 months after insertion, were run in a hip joint simulator. The frictional torques were found to correlate with the location of the wear areas in the cups, and equatorial contact, resulting from small geometric irregularities on the head or in the cup, was shown to produce extremely high values of frictional torque. Walker and Gold speculated that equatorial contact in McKee–Farrar prostheses could produce loosening in some patients.

Weightman et al. (1972, 1973) used the hip joint simulator shown in Fig. 3.9 to compare the friction and wear characteristics of three widely used total hip prostheses. The prostheses were embedded in polymethylmethacrylate in the machine at the compound angles found in the body. A suitably profiled cam and mechanical linkage provided a flexion–extension cycle to the femoral component while a second cam, acting through a parallelogram loading frame, applied a fluctuating load with a peak value of 3·5 kN to the acetabular component. The loading arrangement was such that the acetabular cup was allowed to 'float' on top of the femoral head. The instrumentation of the simulator consisted of a strain gauge network on the vertical members of the loading frame and a force transducer–load cell combination attached to the acetabular component a fixed distance from the centre of rotation of the femoral head. This arrangement allowed a continuous recording of frictional torque and load.

In the first series of tests the friction and lubrication of a 32 mm diameter cobalt–chromium alloy against high density polyethylene Charnley–Müller prosthesis and a 41 mm diameter all-cobalt–chromium alloy McKee–Farrar prosthesis were studied and compared. Coefficients of friction were calculated by converting frictional torque readings to tangential friction force values at the

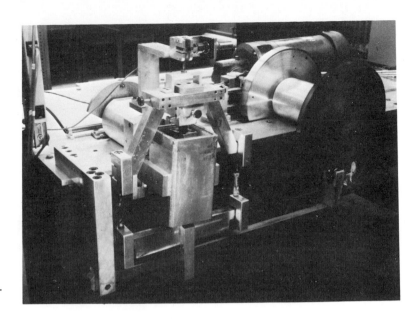

Figure 3.9.
The hip joint simulator used by Weightman et al. (1972, 1973).

rubbing surface and dividing by the applied load (i.e. assuming polar contact). Tests were conducted with four different lubricants: bovine serum, bovine synovial fluid, human serum albumin and 0·155 molar veronate buffer.

Under a load of 2·5 kN serum, serum albumin and synovial fluid gave almost identical coefficients of friction with the all-metal prosthesis (0·12–0·13) whereas veronate buffer produced a value of approximately 0·22. With the metal-to-plastic prosthesis, serum and synovial fluid produced similar values (approximately 0·06–0·07) while those for serum albumin and veronate buffer were somewhat higher (0·10–0·12).

Tests under different loads with serum as lubricant showed that the coefficient of friction of both types of prosthesis decreased with increasing load (Fig. 3.10). In order to investigate this character-

Figure 3.10.
Coefficient of friction versus load for Charnley–Müller (metal-on-plastic) and McKee–Farrar (metal-on-metal) total hip replacements (Weightman et al., 1972).

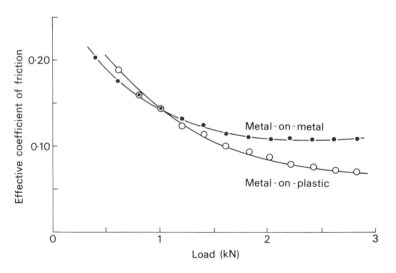

istic, further tests were conducted without lubricant so that a comparison of the two sets of results would indicate the effect of the lubricant. Under dry conditions the relationships between frictional force and load for the metal-to-metal and the metal-to-plastic prostheses were found to be

$$F = 0.55L \quad \text{and} \quad F = 0.85L^{0.83}$$

respectively.

These relationships can be explained by the plastic deformation of contacting metal asperities giving a friction force directly proportional to load for the metal–metal joints, and the partly elastic and partly plastic deformation of polyethylene asperities leading to a relationship of the form

$$F = k.L^n$$

for the metal–plastic points (see section 1.1 of this chapter).

When lubricated, the frictional force of the metal–metal prosthesis was equal to a term directly proportional to load plus a constant; that is,

$$F = 0.084L + 12.5$$

Close agreement with experimental data for the lubricated metal–plastic prosthesis was obtained by assuming that the frictional force was equal to a term proportional to load to the power 0.83 (same as dry) plus a constant. This relationship was

$$F = 0.11L^{0.83} + 22$$

Weightman et al. postulated that the load-dependent term in the two equations described the material–material interaction while the constant term was associated with the liquid. The fact that the fluid term was constant with increasing load suggested a constant thickness. An estimate of the thickness based on geometry and fluid viscosity indicated an extremely thin film inconsistent with the force resulting from viscous shear of fluid layers. It was concluded that the fluid component of the friction force was probably due to the shearing of large molecules making up a boundary lubricant layer.

In their second paper these authors compared the friction and wear characteristics of Charnley, Charnley–Müller, and McKee–Farrar prostheses. Two examples of each type of replacement were run in the simulator at 30 cycles per minute for 1000 hours with bovine serum as lubricant. Coefficients of friction under a static load of 2.5 kN were monitored throughout the tests and the radial depth wear of the acetabular cups was measured after 500 and 1000 hours with a specially designed instrument. This wear gauge compared the radial depth of the cups at 120 points before and after periods in the simulator.

Table 3.1 gives a summary of the results. The maximum radial depths of wear for the Charnley, Charnley–Müller, and McKee–Farrar prostheses were 0.15, 0.075 and 0.013 mm respectively, although in all three cases the wear during the second 500 hours of the test was less than during the first 500 hours. Since 1000 hours in the simulator at 30 cycles per minute (1.8 million cycles) is approximately equal to one year's normal *in vivo* activity, the wear results indicated that none of the prostheses tested is likely to fail as the result of the femoral head wearing through the acetabular cup.

The Charnley and Charnley–Müller prostheses (both metal against high density polyethylene) gave essentially the same coefficient of friction (0·05) although in the case of the Charnley–Müller prostheses it took some 400 hours for the values to fall from approximately 0·10. There was no such evidence of a 'running-in' process with the McKee–Farrar joints; in fact the coefficient of friction increased gradually from 0·10 to 0·13 throughout the test for one of these prostheses while for the other the value stayed at 0·14.

Commenting on the significance of these measured coefficients of friction Weightman et al. concluded that, since for a given load the frictional torque in the plane of flexion–extension is proportional to the product of the measured coefficient of friction and the radius of the head, the McKee–Farrar prosthesis, with the largest coefficient of friction and the largest diameter head, produces the largest frictional torque, while the Charnley prosthesis, with the smallest diameter head, produces the lowest. Since the areas of contact in the two tested McKee–Farrar prostheses were polar, the authors speculated that the frictional torque in these prostheses would gradually increase with further wear as the wear areas spread out towards the equator of the cups. The gradual increase in measured coefficient of friction from 0·10 to 0·13 during the test of one of the McKee–Farrar prostheses was thought to reflect this trend. On the basis of these laboratory tests, the authors therefore concluded that the incidence of acetabular cup loosening should be least with the Charnley prosthesis and greatest with the McKee–Farrar prosthesis.

The coefficients of friction quoted above were measured while the prostheses were running. Since the force necessary to initiate sliding is greater than that required to maintain sliding, Simon et al. (1975) studied the effect of static friction (or stiction) on the frictional torques (and therefore the stresses at the cement interfaces) generated in total hip replacements. Using the hip joint simulator previously described (see Fig 3.9) with serum, synovial fluid and veronate buffer as lubricants, the effect of different pre-motion loading times and loads on the static frictional torques of a McKee–Farrar and a Charnley–Müller prosthesis were measured. The results showed that the static friction increased only after relatively long stationary periods under high load, and the authors therefore concluded that under physiological conditions 'stiction–friction' differed little from dynamic friction in both metal-on-metal and metal-on-plastic prostheses.

Table 3.1 Hip Joint Simulator Results (Weightman et al. 1972)

	Charnley (22 mm dia. head)		Charnley–Müller (32 mm dia. head)		McKee–Farrar (41 mm dia. head)	
	No. 1	No. 2	No. 1	No. 2	No. 1	No. 2
Maximum radial depth wear in cup after 500 hours (mm)	0·110	0·130	0·063	0·050	0·010	0·013
Maximum radial depth wear in cup after 1000 hours (mm)	0·150	0·150	0·075	0·075	0·013	0·013
Effective coefficient of friction (under a static load of 2·5 kN)	0·05	0·06	0·04	0·06	0·13	0·14

Gold and Walker (1974) used a hip joint simulator to study the effect of head diameter, surface finish, sphericity, and clearance between head and cup, on the friction and wear of metal-on-plastic total hip replacements. Various metal femoral components (Charnley, Trapezoidal and Müller) were supplied by the manufacturers and acetabular components were made out of uhmw polyethylene and polytetrafluorethylene in the authors' workshops. Each combination was run for 30 hours under a fluctuating load (2 kN maximum) and wear was measured as the weight of particles filtered out of the distilled water lubricant.

Frictional torque measurements with uhmw polyethylene showed that torque was directly proportional to head diameter. In wear tests with polyethylene the variations in wear rate between the different prostheses (with different head size, surface finish, sphericity, and roughness) were no more than would be expected in repeated wear experiments (with no variables changed), so that it was difficult to draw any conclusions as to the effect (if any) of these variables upon wear rate. However, a surface roughness of 0·05–0·1 μm (root mean square) appeared to produce greater wear than a surface roughness of 0·05–0·075 μm. A second finding from this series of tests was that a stainless steel Charnley prosthesis and a cobalt–chromium alloy Charnley prosthesis produced approximately the same amount of wear so that, within the limits of the experiment, the type of alloy appeared to have no effect.

In tests with PTFE the amounts of wear were greater than with polyethylene but again the differences between prostheses were not great. However, the results seemed to indicate that:

(1) 28 mm diameter heads produced slightly less cup wear than either 22 mm or 32 mm diameter heads;

(2) variations in clearance between heads and cups (i.e. differences in radii) of between 100 and 500 μm had little or no effect on wear rate;

(3) lack of sphericity of up to 10 μm (the maximum tested) had little or no effect on wear rate; and

(4) the wear rate increased slightly when the surface roughness approached 0·1 μm.

Boutin (1972) discussed the mechanical and chemical properties of pure dense aluminium oxide (Al_2O_3) ceramic and reported the results of simulator wear tests on a total hip prosthesis with bearing surfaces of this material. The advantages of the material were listed as extreme hardness, excellent compressive strength, chemical inertness, and tissue acceptability. The hip prosthesis consisted of a ceramic femoral head attached to a metallic femoral shaft with epoxy cement, and a ceramic acetabular cup. The simulator ran at 1 cycle per second under a load of 1 kN with saline as lubricant, and wear measurements were made every 300 hours. There was 10 μm wear on the head during the first 300 hours, 3 μm wear between 300 and 600 hours, and zero wear between 600 and 2 100 hours, the end of the test. No wear was found in the acetabular cups. Surface roughness measurements showed that the head became smoother during the test. The surface finish improved from between 0·15 and 0·3 μm (centre line average) to 0·1 μm during the first 300 hours, to 0·06 μm after 600 hours, and then showed no change.

At first sight the correlation between wear rate and improving surface finish suggests that the wear process was simply the removal of the original surface asperities, and that when the surface finish had improved to 0·06 μm (after 600 hours) the wear process ceased. A closer look at the data shows this not to be the case. The original surface had a peak-to-trough height of approximately 1·75 μm. If the asperities were totally removed to form a perfectly flat surface this would only account for 1·75 μm wear. The fact that Boutin measured a total depth of wear of 13 μm shows that something more than a polishing process was involved.

Although Boutin and many other workers have referred to the excellent chemical inertness of aluminium oxide ceramic, Schmittgrund, Kenner and Brown (1972) found that the material loses strength when soaked in saline solution or implanted into the soft tissue of animals. There is, therefore, the possibility of degradative wear of this material in the body.

Most of the tests with joint simulators have aimed at studying the performance of total hip replacements in hip joint simulators. As far as the present author is aware the only published work describing simulator tests of total knee replacements is that of Swanson, Freeman and Heath (1973). Shiers and Walldius' all-cobalt–chromium hinged total knee prostheses were run in a simulator under constant load (0·89 kN) with Ringer's solution as lubricant. Significant quantities of particulate wear debris were produced and the abrasive wear scratches on the hinge pins of the simulator-tested prostheses were shown to be similar to those on a pin from a prosthesis removed from a patient.

To date no results of simulator tests of hingeless metal-on-plastic total knee replacements have been published. Some of the designers of such prostheses have carried out simulator tests but have not published the results (for example, Swanson, personal communication); others have based their designs either on the satisfactory performance of high molecular weight polyethylene in total hip replacements or on the results of wear tests with machines of the block-on-disc type previously described (section 2.1 of this chapter).

2.2.2 SUMMARY

Laboratory work with joint simulators indicates that:

(1) Of possible metal-on-metal combinations only cast cobalt–chromium alloy on itself is suitable from a friction and wear point of view. Such prostheses are well lubricated by synovial fluid, the mechanism being boundary lubrication and not fluid film. In order to minimise frictional torque, and hence the possibility of loosening, all-metal total hip prostheses must have a geometry and a degree of sphericity (lack of out-of-roundness) which produces polar contact, and an excellent surface finish. Under these conditions the volumetric rate of wear of all-metal total hip replacements is extremely low.

(2) The frictional torques produced by metal-on-high density polyethylene total hip replacements are lower than those produced by all-cobalt–chromium alloy prostheses, but the volumetric rate of wear (of the polyethylene) is greater. There is very little experimental evidence concerning the optimum head size, surface finish, sphericity, and clearance for metal-on-polyethylene total hip replacements, but what there is suggests that:

(a) the rate of depth wear in the polyethylene cup decreases with increasing head size;

(b) the volumetric rate of wear of the polyethylene is perhaps less with a 28 mm diameter head than with either a 22 mm or a 32 mm diameter head;

(c) the frictional torque produced is directly proportional to head diameter;

(d) the surface finish on the metal head should be better than $0 \cdot 1 \ \mu$m (root mean square);

(e) the rate of wear is affected little by variations in clearance of between 100 and 500 μm between the components and lack of sphericity of up to 10 μm.

(3) Aluminium oxide ceramic appears to be a promising material for the bearing surfaces of total joint replacements. This conclusion is based on the results of only one simulator test and conflicts with the results from disc-on-disc and pin-on-disc wear tests. Clearly, further laboratory investigations are required, particularly into the possibility of degradative wear, before widespread clinical use of the material.

(4) All-cobalt–chromium alloy hinged total knee prostheses produce significant quantities of wear debris.

2.3 The Examination of Removed Prostheses

2.3.1 REVIEW OF THE LITERATURE

Swikert and Johnson (1971) examined two cast cobalt–chromium alloy McKee–Farrar total hip prostheses removed after 1–2 years of service. Roundness measurements highlighted the problem of the fit between the head and the cup. On the two prostheses examined the area of contact between head and cup was reduced to approximately 50 per cent of the possible area, and was situated towards the rim (equator) of the cups. Examination of the worn areas showed voids resulting from the shearing of adhesively formed junctions and deep scratches produced by the abrasive action of the adhesively formed wear particles. Although wear was thought to have been initiated by adhesion, abrasion was considered the principal source of wear debris.

Walker and Gold (1971) examined the areas of wear in 10 McKee–Farrar prostheses removed from patients between 3 and 18 months after insertion. Surface profile traces and scanning electron microscopy of new and used acetabular cups showed that the original asperities had been removed during a running-in process and that surface scratches had then been produced by the resulting particles (three-body abrasive wear).

Weightman et al. (1973) compared simulator-tested McKee–Farrar, Charnley–Müller and Charnley total hip prostheses with the same types of prostheses removed from patients. With each type the same wear mechanisms were found to have occurred *in vitro* and *in vivo*. The metallic cups of the McKee–Farrar hips contained abrasive scratches thought to be the result of the abrasive action of wear debris produced by adhesion. Wear areas in the Charnley and Charnley–Müller polyethylene cups had a generally polished appearance but wear scratches were present. The polished appearance was thought to have been produced by the localised plastic flow of asperities on the original machined surface. The scratches were thought to be indicative of a combination of abrasive and brittle fracture wear. Brittle fracture wear (section 1.2) is characterised by cracks running perpendicularly across the width of wear tracks and into the material perpendicular to the surface. On replicas of the surface viewed in a scanning electron microscope (Fig. 3.11) the cracks appeared as thin wafers of replicating tape protruding above the ridge of the wear tracks. The occurrence of brittle fracture wear in uhmw polyethylene was surprising since, under normal conditions, the material does not behave in a brittle manner. One of the possible explanations discussed by Weightman et al. was chemical degradation of the polymer, by synovial fluid in the patients and serum in the simulator.

Figure 3.11.
Brittle fracture wear in a polyethylene acetabular cup (replica).

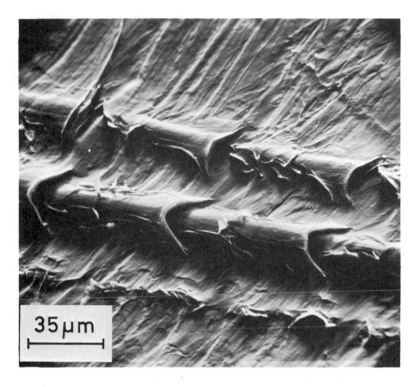

35 μm

Walker and Gold (1973) studied 11 McKee–Farrar and 4 Charnley total hip prostheses (removed between 6 months and 2 years after insertion) with light microscopy, surface profile tracings, and scanning electron microscopy of originals and replicas. Only a very small amount of material had been removed from the McKee–Farrar components. Examination under a light microscope showed two distinctly different types of wear area. In the first, mild to severe scratching had apparently been produced by the adhesive wear of original high spots followed by abrasion. The second type of wear area had a dull appearance under a light microscope with only a few visible scratches. The authors considered these areas to have undergone an 'advanced' form of wear consisting of a much more 'refined' adhesive or abrasive mechanism. Contact areas in the Charnley prostheses covered a large part of the cup surfaces. Most of the contact area in each cup was polished, but some regions presented a dull or matt texture. In the scanning electron microscope the polished areas were seen to contain abrasive scratches 1–5 μm in width and ripples of 0·5–1 μm pitch perpendicular to the scratches.

Parallel to the ripples were small cracks a few micrometres long. Both rippling and cracking were thought to be the result of the to and fro stretching of the plastic surface. The dull areas to the side of the polished regions had an extremely rough 'shredded' appearance, the shreds being up to 5 μm long. Apparently the shreds had been caused by the localised stretching of the plastic surface.

Since the size of the abrasive scratches and shreds did not correlate with the surface irregularities on the metal head (0·1 μm polishing scratches) Walker and Gold speculated that the surface roughness of the head played an insignificant part in the wear process, and that the tensile and fatigue properties of the polyethylene were of primary importance.

To date there have been no reports in the literature giving details of the examination of removed metal-on-polyethylene total knee replacements. However, Radin et al. (1974) and Bullough et al. (1976) have commented that the abrasive wear produced by methacrylate particles trapped between the bearing surfaces has been a significant problem. These authors speculate that the concave tibial components act as collection basins. Experiences with the ICLH total knee replacement (Freeman, unpublished data) only partly supports these comments. Methacrylate particles have been found embedded in removed polyethylene tibial components but it is unclear whether or not this has produced a significantly increased wear rate. The cement particles have certainly damaged the surfaces of the components but they would have produced three-body abrasive wear only if they ploughed through the polyethylene. If they became embedded immediately they entered the joint, any abrasive action would have been prevented.

2.3.2 DISCUSSION

The examination of removed all-cobalt–chromium alloy total hip replacements has shown that wear is initiated by adhesion and continued by the abrasive action of the adhesively formed wear particles (three-body abrasive wear). As Swikert and Johnson (1971) point out, improvements in the roundness and surface finish of the components might reduce the incidence of adhesive wear and the provision of crossed grooves in the bearing surfaces might reduce the abrasive wear rate by allowing the abrasive particles to escape from between the surfaces.

The mechanism of polyethylene wear in metal-on-polyethylene total hip replacements is less clear but appears to be a combination of abrasion and either brittle fracture wear or fatigue wear (or both). The abrasive wear cannot be explained by the surface roughness of the metal head and therefore appears to be three-body abrasive wear, the particles being produced by adhesion, brittle fracture or fatigue, or extraneous material.

In a recent paper, Crugnola et al. (1976) discussed the phenomenon of environment-enhanced brittle fracture of polyethylene and emphasised the importance of molecular weight distribution rather than average molecular weight. Other things being equal, the tendency for brittle fracture to occur in a particular environment depends not on the average molecular weight of the polyethylene but on the amount of low molecular weight material present; the greater the amount of low molecular weight material, the greater the chance of brittle fracture and hence of brittle fracture wear.

These workers studied the molecular weight distributions in uhmw polyethylene acetabular cups obtained from six different manufacturers. They found significant amounts (10–25 per cent) of low molecular weight polymer in samples taken from the interior of all six components. Five of the six samples taken from the bearing surfaces of each cup contained between 5 and 15 per cent low molecular weight material while the remaining sample contained 75 per cent. Although this work does not establish the occurrence of brittle fracture wear in uhmw polyethylene components *in vivo*, it does indicate the theoretical possibility.

Information about the mechanism of polyethylene wear in hingeless total knee replacements is sadly lacking, although limited clinical evidence suggests that three-body abrasive wear produced by methacrylate particles may be a problem. If this should prove to be the case, laboratory tests with knee joint simulators should be used to study possible ways of reducing the wear rate. Medial-lateral grooves in the surface of polyethylene tibial components, for example, might arrest the action of the abrasive particles.

2.4 Clinical Results

2.4.1 REVIEW OF THE LITERATURE

Low wear rates and the intrinsic difficulty of measuring wear *in vivo* mean that wear rates can only be measured with any reasonable degree of accuracy over relatively long periods of time. This is one reason why very few of the published clinical studies of total joint replacements have dealt specifically with the problem of wear.

Only Charnley has systematically measured wear rates in the body. Charnley first used polytetrafluorethylene (PTFE, Fluon or Teflon) for the plastic component of his total hip replacement. The wear rate of this material against a 22 mm diameter femoral head was measured from x-rays and removed specimens and found to be between 2·4 and 3·6 mm per year (Charnley, Kamangar and Longfield 1969). When Charnley started to use high molecular weight polyethylene sockets a semicircular reference wire was incorporated in the outer circumference so that wear could be measured as loss of concentricity with the head on anteroposterior radiographs. Since then periodic follow-up reviews have provided measurements of the wear of this material in the body. Of the 72 cases studied after 4 and 5 years, 37 had wear of approximately 1 mm while the remaining 35 had no detectable wear (Charnley 1970). This low wear rate during the first few years in the body was later confirmed by direct measurement of a number of cups obtained at necropsy, which showed an average wear rate of 0·13 mm per year (Charnley 1971). Still later results, obtained from x-rays, showed that the low initial rate of wear was maintained for up to 9 and 10 years (Charnley and Cupic 1973). Of the 72 cases studied, 62 (86 per cent) had worn 1·5 mm or less, with an average of 0·09 mm per year; the remaining 10 (14 per cent) had worn up to 4 mm, with an average of 0·3 mm per year. The average wear rate for the 72 cases combined was 0·12 mm per year. In this study wear was measured from a single x-ray by subtracting the narrowest measurement between the head and wire marker from the widest measurement in the non-weight-bearing area, and dividing by 2. Because of criticisms that this method could produce large errors, a second study of the 9- and 10-year results was made (Charnley and Halley 1975) in which wear was measured by comparing the thickness of the plastic in the most recent radiograph with the thickness in the immediately postoperative film at the same point. The results of this second study were in close agreement with those of the previous study. It was found that 68 per cent of cases had worn 1·5 mm or less, while the remaining 32 per cent had worn up to 4·5 mm in 10 years. In the whole series, the average wear was 1·5 mm over 9 or 10 years (an average wear rate of 0·15 mm per year).

An average wear rate of 0·15 mm per year was also obtained from direct measurements of 26 acetabular cups removed at post-mortem (Charnley 1974).

The variations in wear rate could not be explained by variations in patients' body weight or, apparently, by variations in their physical activity, and were therefore thought to be the result of differences in the quality of the high density polyethylene (Charnley and Cupic 1973).

A particularly interesting finding of the later study (Charnley and Halley 1975) was that the average wear rate during the second 5-year period was approximately 40 per cent lower than that during the first 5 years.

All the above results were obtained with a 22 mm diameter femoral head. In the 1971 paper referred to above, Charnley listed the advantages of this relatively small head as being a reduced volume of wear debris and a lower frictional torque. The greater cup wall thickness was considered to compensate for the admittedly higher rate of depth wear.

Of the other possible polymeric materials for use in total joint replacements the clinical experience with polyester is worthy of note. In 1968 Weber introduced a new design of total hip replacement, the Trunnion Bearing prosthesis, with a plastic ball bearing against a cobalt–chromium alloy acetabular cup. A cylindrical peg on a cobalt–chromium alloy femoral stem fitted into a cylindrical hole in the plastic ball so that the prosthesis contained two bearings: one cylindrical and one spherical (Weber 1970). After more than 2 years, balls of AP3 and AP4 polyester, which had been removed because of late loosening, showed no measurable change in diameter although the surfaces had become highly polished (Weber and Semlitsch 1972). However, Weber and Stühmer (1976) reported that the high incidence of loosening in the 1 000 polyester prostheses inserted between 1968 and 1972 could be attributed to the foreign body reaction to abraded polyester, and that the prostheses were being converted to a cobalt–chromium alloy ball against a polyethylene cup.

Since laboratory tests (Scales 1972; and see section 2.1.1 of this chapter) have shown that polyester is liable to hydrolysis and that this disastrously affects its wear resistance, it seems almost certain that chemical degradation was a major factor in the clinical failure of the material. However, an important contributing factor could well have been the use of a polymeric ball (convex) and a metallic cup (concave). As has already been shown (see section 2.1.1 of this chapter), such a configuration will result in greater wear of the polymer than a metal ball in a polymer cup, and this will be particularly true in the presence of a degrading environment.

Clinical experience with ultra-high molecular weight polyethylene has confirmed that this material has sufficient wear resistance for use in total hip replacements. The apparent decrease in depth wear rate with time is particularly encouraging and suggests that metal-on-polyethylene total hip replacements will perform satisfactorily for considerably longer than 10 years. That is, whatever the wear mechanisms, the wear rate appears to be sufficiently low to ensure a considerable life before the femoral head wears through the acetabular cup.

This optimistic forecast is clouded by three considerations. Firstly, there is considerable variation in the clinically observed wear rates with a small percentage of cases wearing at up to three times the average rate. Further research is needed to explain this variation since in the Charnley prosthesis, for example, a continued depth wear rate of 0·45 mm per year would give only a 20-year life before the femoral head wore through the acetabular cup. One possibility is that the variation results from differences in the fraction of low molecular weight material present in the polyethylene, and that these produce different rates of brittle fracture wear in the body (see section 2.3.2 of this chapter). If this should prove to be the case the remedy would appear to be relatively simple in principle, although perhaps less simple in practice.

Secondly, failure of total joint replacements may result from the body's reaction to a build-up of wear debris in the tissue surrounding the implant. Such failures are known to have occurred with PTFE and polyester. While there is little evidence of a similar reaction to polyethylene wear debris in the hip over a 10-year period, the possibility that a build-up of debris over 15 or 20 years may lead to failure should not be overlooked. The rate of volumetric wear of polyethylene in total hip replacements depends to a large extent on the size of the femoral head, and the effect of the design of the prosthesis on the rate of production of wear debris is discussed in the following section of this chapter. However, it should be recognised that even if the volumetric wear rate of polyethylene is minimised this may not prevent failure over a long period of time (see Chapter 4).

Thirdly, this forecast is based on wear measurements made on a fairly homogeneous group of elderly and handicapped patients treated in one hospital by a technique probably more closely controlled than is usual. Hips (and other joints) are now being replaced in younger and more active patients, and the effects on wear rates of the higher stresses presumably imposed by these patients are unknown.

The situation with regard to metal-on-polyethylene replacements for other joints such as the knee or ankle is far more uncertain. As previously stated there is a paucity of data on the wear behaviour of such prostheses, and it does not necessarily follow that the wear behaviour of high molecular weight polyethylene will be the same, for example, in knee prostheses as it is in hip prostheses.

3 THE USE OF WEAR THEORY IN THE DESIGN OF TOTAL JOINT REPLACEMENTS

In many ways the design of engineering bearings so as to minimise wear is more of an art than a science. One reason for this is that the lack of a full understanding of the complex mechanisms of wear makes it impossible to predict, from purely theoretical considerations, the nature and magnitude of the wear process which will occur under a particular set of conditions. At best, designing against wear is an empirical science relying heavily on laboratory experiments and practical experience. Unfortunately, the wear rate of any material is extremely sensitive to operating conditions and it can be dangerous to extrapolate from one situation to another. The use of polytetrafluorethylene (PTFE) in total hip replacements provides a good example of this; the wear rate of this material in the body proved to be many time that predicted on the basis of laboratory tests and general engineering experience.

Another difficulty faced by the bearing designer is that factors completely outside his control can make any calculations meaningless. For example, the big-end bearings in a motor car engine will be destroyed if the car owner does not ensure an adequate supply of oil. Similarly, the designer of artificial human joints cannot include in his calculations the effect of the orthopaedic surgeon leaving bone cement between the bearing surfaces.

In spite of these and other difficulties it would seem foolish totally to ignore the existing theory of wear when designing joint replacements. In most cases an imperfect estimate is likely to be better than pure guesswork. On the basis of this premise, the following sections of this chapter illustrate how the basic wear equation

$$v = \frac{c.L.x}{p} \qquad \text{(see section 1.3)}$$

can be used to predict the effect of various design parameters on the wear behaviour of certain types of artificial joint. Even though a number of assumptions are made during the analysis it is suggested that the resulting conclusions, concerning the relative advantages and disadvantages of different designs of artificial joint, are valid until either a more accurate analysis or direct clinical experience contradicts them.

The vast majority of total joint replacements are now metal-on-polymer combinations and virtually all of these are essentially balls in sockets or rollers in troughs. The following sections, dealing with metal-on-polymer total hips and hingeless metal-on-polymer total knees, therefore illustrate the basic design considerations for a large number of total joint replacements.

3.1 The Effect of Femoral Head Size on the Wear of Metal-on-Polymer Total Hip Replacements

3.1.1 MATHEMATICAL ANALYSIS

In the case of metal-on-polymer ball-and-socket joints such as the hip, one of the most important design variables as far as wear is concerned is the diameter of the femoral head. The basic wear equation can be used to indicate how femoral head size might be expected to influence the volume of polymeric wear debris produced per year, the rate at which the femoral head wears through the polymer cup, and the time taken for the head to wear completely through the cup.

Since the sliding distance per unit time is directly proportional to the femoral head diameter for a fixed range of movement, the load across the joint (L) is independent of head size, and the hardness of the surface being worn away (p) is a property of the material, the volume of wear debris produced per year should be directly proportional to head diameter. That is, the basic wear equation becomes

$$v_t = C.d \qquad \ldots(7)$$

where v_t is the volume of debris produced per year (mm³ per year),

C is a constant, and

d is the femoral head diameter (mm).

This equation assumes that the wear coefficient in the original wear equation (c) does not vary with head diameter; that is, it does not vary with nominal contact pressure. Although this is probably not strictly true, it appears to be a reasonable assumption provided the nominal contact pressure does not approach the yield stress of the polymer, and increased rubbing speeds do not significantly increase the temperature at the contact surfaces. To support the equation there is the clinical experience with polytetrafluorethylene (PTFE) (Charnley, Kamangar and Longfield 1969) which showed an approximately linear increase in volume of wear debris produced per year with increasing femoral head diameter in the range 22–44 mm.

The volume of wear debris produced per year will be equal to the product of depth of wear per year (penetration into the cup) and the cross-sectional area of the femoral head, so that

$$v_t = h_t . \frac{\pi d^2}{4} \quad \text{mm}^3 \text{ per year} \qquad \ldots(8)$$

where h_t is the depth of wear per year (mm per year).

Combining equations (7) and (8) gives

$$h_t = \frac{B}{d} \qquad \ldots(9)$$

where B is a new constant.

This equation indicates that the rate of depth wear is inversely proportional to head diameter, so that the smaller the femoral head the greater the rate of depth wear. At first sight this suggests that joints with small femoral heads will wear out faster than joints with large femoral heads. However, for a fixed outside diameter of acetabular cup, the smaller the head diameter the greater the wall thickness. The time taken for the femoral head to wear through the cup is therefore obtained by dividing the wall thickness by the rate of depth wear. If the inner and outer surfaces of the cup are concentric, the wall thickness is given by

$$\text{Wall thickness} = \tfrac{1}{2}(D-d) \qquad \ldots(10)$$

where D is the outside diameter.

Dividing this expression by the rate of depth wear (equation 9), gives

$$\text{Time to penetration} = \tfrac{1}{2}(D-d)\frac{d}{B} \quad \text{years} \quad \ldots(11)$$

It can be shown mathematically that whatever the value of the constant B, for any given outside diameter (D) the time to penetration will be a maximum if the femoral head diameter (d) is one-half the outside diameter.

Ideally, artificial hip joints should produce the smallest possible volume of wear debris per year and the femoral head should not wear through the cup within the remaining life of the patient. Since the equations for volume of debris per year and time to penetration (equations 7 and 11) both contain unknown constants (C and B), they cannot be evaluated. For this reason the only conclusions that can be drawn from them are that:

(1) if wear debris is likely to cause problems, the femoral head diameter should be as small as possible in order to minimise the volume of debris produced per year; and

(2) if there is a danger of the femoral head wearing through the cup within the remaining life of the patient, the diameter of the femoral head should be half the outside diameter of the cup which itself should be as large as possible.

The analysis above is relevant to all total hip replacements which have a femoral head made out of a hard (non-wearing) material and an acetabular cup made out of a softer (wearing) material. Although the general discussion cannot be extended, in the special case of total hip replacements with polyethylene cups clinical experience can be used to calculate the value of the constants in the equations. This means that both the volume of polyethylene wear debris produced per year by any size of femoral head and the time it will take for any size femoral head to wear through any size of acetabular cap can be estimated.

Clinical experience of the Charnley prosthesis over a 10-year period (Charnley and Halley 1975) has shown an average rate of depth wear of 0·15 mm per year. Using this figure together with the diameter of the Charnley femoral head (22 mm) in equation (9) gives a value of 3·3 for the constant B. Substituting this value of B into equation (11) gives

$$\text{Time to penetration} = \frac{(D-d)d}{6\cdot6} \quad \text{years} \quad \ldots(12)$$

This equation can now be used to estimate the time it will take for any size femoral head to wear through a polyethylene cup of any outside diameter.

If the value of 0·15 mm per year for the rate of depth wear of the Charnley prosthesis and a diameter of 22 mm are substituted into equation (8), the volume of wear debris produced per year by the Charnley prosthesis is estimated to be 57·0 mm³. Putting this value into equation (7) yields a figure of 2·6 for the constant C. Equation (7) therefore becomes

$$v_t = 2\cdot6\,.\,d \qquad \ldots(13)$$

and this can now be used to estimate the volume of polyethylene wear debris produced per year by any size femoral head.

Figure 3.12 shows how the volume of polyethylene wear debris produced per year and the time for the head to wear through the cup vary with femoral head size, as predicted by equations (13) and

(12) respectively. The three curves in Fig. 3.12b are for three different outside diameters of cup, covering the range currently used in total hip prostheses. For reference purposes, points representing the predicted wear behaviour of two commonly used total hip replacements—the Charnley type with a 22 mm diameter femoral head and a 40 mm diameter cup (point 1), and the Charnley–Müller type with a 32 mm diameter head and a 50 mm cup (point 2)—are included in the graphs.

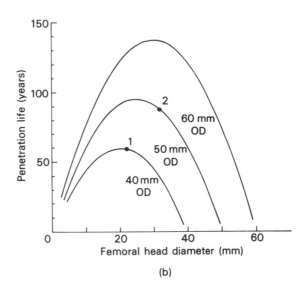

Figure 3.12.
The effect of femoral head size on (a) the volumetric wear rate of polyethylene, and (b) the penetration life of different size acetabular cups. Point 1 represents the Charnley prosthesis and point 2 the Charnley–Müller.

Figure 3.12b clearly illustrates that for a given outside diameter of cup, the analysis predicts a maximum penetration time if the femoral head diameter is half the cup outside diameter. It is also clear that even an acetabular cup with an outside diameter as small as 40 mm should have sufficient wall thickness for at least 50 years' clinical use if the femoral head diameter is between 12 and 28 mm. An acetabular cup with an outside diameter of 50 mm should have sufficient wall thickness if the femoral head is between 8 and 42 mm in diameter.

77

Figure 3.12a illustrates how the volume of polyethylene wear debris is expected to vary with head size. The increasing volume of debris with increasing head size together with the prediction that the time to penetration of a 60 mm outside diameter cup is a maximum when the femoral head diameter is 30 mm indicates that, from the point of view of wear, there is no virtue in having femoral heads larger than 30 mm in diameter. Above this size the penetration life of the prosthesis decreases and the rate of production of wear particles increases.

In fact, there seems little benefit (again from the point of view of wear) in having a femoral head diameter as large as 30 mm, since the penetration time of such a combination is predicted to be 136 years. If the head size were 25 mm, the penetration time would still be more than 130 years and the rate of production of wear debris would be reduced from 78 to 65 mm³ per year (17 per cent).

Figure 3.12 suggests that metal-against-polyethylene total hip replacements should have a femoral head diameter less than 20 mm. Such a prosthesis would be expected to have penetration times well over 50 years and low rates of wear debris production. Even from pure engineering considerations, however, this situation could lead to problems since the nominal contact stress increases by a square power as the diameter decreases. Any proposed reduction in femoral head size below the minimum at present found to be satisfactory would require exhaustive tests to confirm that the wear coefficient (c), and hence the wear rate, was not increased by the increase in nominal contact stress.

There is another engineering consideration which places a lower limit on femoral head size. This is concerned with the effect of head size on the range of motion of the joint and the decreasing range of motion as the head wears into the cup. The range of motion of an artificial hip joint is a complex problem in three-dimensional geometry, involving rotation about three mutually perpendicular axes. However, a crude assessment of the problem can be made with a relatively simple two-dimensional analysis. Figure 3.13a gives details of the model; a spherical femoral head with diameter D, a cylindrical neck with a diameter d, and a hemispherical acetabular cup. It is clear that the range of motion in the plane of the diagram is limited by contact between the neck and the edge of the cup. Figure 3.13b illustrates the fact that as the head wears into the cup the range of motion is gradually reduced.

Two points follow from these diagrams. Firstly, the range of motion of an unworn hip replacement depends to a certain extent on the ratio of head diameter to neck diameter. Other factors being equal (e.g. the angle subtended by the cup), the larger this ratio the larger the range of motion. (If the head were the same diameter as the neck, the range of motion would be zero.) It follows that for a given neck diameter the larger the femoral head the greater the range of motion. This general conclusion is supported by laboratory measurements of the various ranges of motion of different types of total hip replacements (Amstutz et al. 1975). For example, with zero abduction, Charnley, Müller and McKee–Farrar total hips were found to be capable of 80°, 96° and 105° flexion respectively, and internal rotations at 90° flexion were 0°, 6° and 14° respectively.

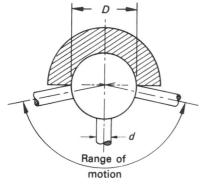

(a) Unworn cup

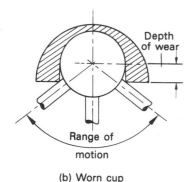

(b) Worn cup

Figure 3.13.
The effect of cup wear on the range of motion of total hip replacements.

Secondly, since the rate of depth wear is predicted to be inversely proportional to head diameter (equation 9), the rate at which the range of motion is reduced as the cup wears is greater for smaller heads. In general, therefore, the smaller the femoral head, the smaller the initial range of motion of the joint and the faster the reduction in range of motion throughout its life. Since movement will be limited by impingement between the femoral neck and the acetabular cup, prostheses with a small head might, in clinical practice, be expected to display a diminishing range of movement, an increased incidence of loosening, or an increased (but possibly undetectable) incidence of spontaneously reducing subluxations with the passage of time.

3.1.2 SUMMARY AND CONCLUSIONS

With polyethylene acetabular cups of outside diameter between 40 and 60 mm, a wide range of femoral head sizes can be used without the danger of the head wearing through the cup within the remaining life of the patient. In terms of wear, the choice of femoral head size appears to lie between a relatively low volumetric rate of wear and a relatively restricted range of motion on the one hand, and a relatively high volumetric rate of wear and a relatively large range of motion on the other.

Until there is a full understanding of the biological effects of a gradual build-up of polyethylene wear debris it is clearly desirable to minimise the volume of debris produced per year, especially in younger patients. On the other hand, by reducing the range of motion to such an extent that the femoral neck might eventually impinge on the acetabular cup, a high rate of depth wear could lead to loosening of the joint. Although the theoretical analysis has highlighted the various effects of different femoral head sizes, the final decision therefore has to be made on the basis of practical experience. Only further clinical experience will show whether the volume of polyethylene wear debris or a restricted range of motion will be the most important factor limiting the use of existing total hip replacements.

3.2 The Wear of Hingeless Total Knee Replacements

3.2.1 MATHEMATICAL ANALYSIS

Most existing metal-against-polyethylene hingeless knee replacements are essentially: (1) metal rollers in non-conforming troughs of polyethylene; (2) twin metal rollers in non-conforming troughs of polyethylene; (3) metal rollers in conforming troughs of polyethylene; or (4) twin metal rollers in conforming troughs of polyethylene. If these basic designs are simplified as shown in Fig. 3.14, all four may be considered as rollers in conforming troughs, with angles of lap (the angle produced at the centre of the roller by the arc of contact between roller and trough) varying from zero upwards, and different widths. Therefore, by applying the basic wear equation

$$v = \frac{c.L.x}{p}$$

to this one design it is possible to assess the effect of different diameters of roller, different angles of lap, and different widths on the wear behaviour, and hence compare the predicted performance of the four different types of knee. The analysis will also apply to other

Figure 3.14.
Different types of total knee replacements.

Metal

Polyethylene

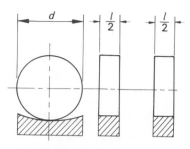

(a) Roller in non-conforming trough

(b) Twin rollers in non-conforming troughs

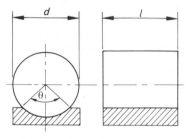

(c) Roller in conforming trough

(d) Twin rollers in conforming troughs

total joint replacements of similar geometry such as the ankle and elbow.

As in the hip joint the load across the joint (L) and the hardness of the polyethylene (p) will not vary with the dimensions of the prosthesis, and if the wear coefficient (c) is assumed to be constant, the volume of wear debris per unit time should be directly proportional to the sliding distance per unit time. Since for a given range of motion the sliding distance per unit time is directly proportional to the diameter (d) of the roller, the basic wear equation can be written

$$v_t = K.d \qquad \qquad \dots(14)$$

where K is a constant.

Thus, according to theory, the volume of wear debris produced per year depends only on the diameter of the roller (or rollers); the larger the diameter, the greater the volume of wear debris.

In a small interval of time, δt, the small volume of polyethylene wear debris produced, δv, will therefore be given by

$$\delta v = K.d.\delta t \qquad \qquad \dots(15)$$

If the depth of wear in this time is δh, then the volume of polyethylene removed will be equal to the area of contact between the roller and trough multiplied by δh. That is,

$$\delta v = \pi d.l.\frac{\theta}{2\pi}.\delta h \qquad \qquad \dots(16)$$

$$= d.\frac{l}{2}.\theta.\delta h$$

where l is the width of the roller, and
θ is the angle of lap in radians.
Equating equations (15) and (16) gives

$$\frac{\delta h}{\delta t} = \frac{2K.d}{d.l.\theta} = \frac{2K}{l.\theta} \qquad \ldots (17)$$

Since $\delta h/\delta t$ is the rate at which the roller will wear into the polyethylene trough (that is, the rate of depth wear), a number of interesting conclusions follow from equation (17):

(1) Since equation (17) does not contain d, the rate of depth wear should be independent of the diameter of the roller.

(2) The rate of depth wear is predicted to be inversely proportional to the angle of lap (θ), so that the larger the angle of lap, the lower will be the rate of depth wear.

(3) As wear progresses, the angle of lap will increase and therefore the rate of depth wear will decrease. Since the maximum possible angle of lap is 180° (π radians), the rate of depth wear will gradually decrease until the arc of contact between the metal and polyethylene is a semicircle. After this the rate of depth wear will remain at the value given by

$$\text{Minimum rate of depth wear} = \frac{K}{\pi.l} = \frac{K'}{l} \qquad \ldots (18)$$

where K' is a new constant.

It should be noted that this represents the theoretical minimum rate of depth wear. In most practical cases an angle of lap of 180° will never occur because the depth of the polyethylene component is less than the radius of the roller.

(4) Equations (17) and (18) indicate that both the rate of depth wear for any given angle of lap and the minimum rate of depth wear when the angle of lap equals 180° are inversely proportional to l, the width of the roller. Clearly the roller should be made as wide as possible in order to minimise the rate of depth wear.

3.2.2 DISCUSSION

The above analysis leads to the general conclusions that, from the point of view of wear, metal-on-polyethylene hingeless knee replacements should have a small diameter to minimise the volume of wear debris produced per year, and a large width and a large angle of lap to minimise the rate of depth wear.

In practice, of course, there are a number of other considerations which place limits on these parameters in hingeless replacements. For example, the required range of motion, the need to remove the minimum amount of bone, and the method of fixation all place lower limits on the diameter and angle of lap. Clearly, hingeless total knee replacements cannot be designed on the basis of the wear analysis alone. Nevertheless, the analysis does provide a basis for the comparison of the theoretical wear behaviour of different designs of total knee prosthesis.

The finding of the wear analysis that the wider the bearing the lower the depth wear rate indicates that the condylar (twin roller) types of replacement (for example, the Geomedic and Polycentric total knees), with their intrinsically smaller widths, will wear into the polyethylene at a faster rate than the full-width roller types of prosthesis (for example, the ICLH total knee).

A second result of the analysis is that the rate of depth wear is inversely proportional to the angle of lap. The general effects of different angles of lap and different widths are summarised in Fig. 3.15. The three curves describe the predicted wear behaviour of different width replacements and the initial depth wear rates of four knee replacements with different combinations of width and angle of lap are shown. The arrows indicate how the rate of depth wear will change as the metal wears into the polyethylene and the angle of lap increases. Unfortunately, until the wear rates of hingeless knee replacements are measured, either in laboratory simulators or from clinical experience, it is impossible to calculate the value of K in equations (14) and (17) and therefore impossible to quantify Fig. 3.15.

Figure 3.15.
The effect of angle of lap and width on the depth wear rate of total knee replacements.

1: Narrow, small angle of lap
2: Wide, small angle of lap
3: Narrow, large angle of lap
4: Wide, large angle of lap

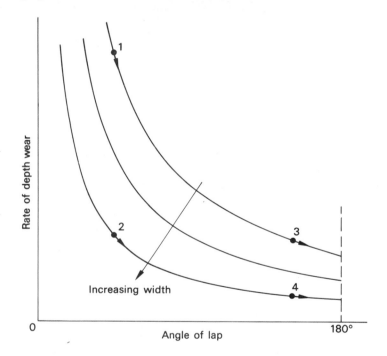

The wear analysis suggests that in non-conforming trough designs the initial rate of depth wear will be infinitely high, since the angle of lap is initially zero. In fact, in these types of knee the polyethylene will deform to produce a conforming trough immediately load is applied, since the initial contact pressure will be infinitely high (zero area of contact) (Seedhom et al. 1972). The angle of lap produced by this deformation will depend on the degree of non-conformity of the two surfaces, but since, in general, the angle of lap produced in an initially non-conforming trough will be less than that in an initial conforming trough, the rate of depth wear is likely to be greater in the former than in the latter.

There is a second reason why the rate of wear is likely to be greater in non-conforming trough than in conforming trough designs. The wear analysis has assumed that the relative motion of the two components of a hingeless total knee replacement is simply rotation about a fixed axis (i.e. the central axis of the femoral roller or rollers). This would appear to be a reasonable assumption in the case of conforming trough designs, since the motion of the joint will be controlled largely by the shape of the articulating surfaces. However, in non-conforming trough designs, and in particular those which tend towards a roller on flat plate configuration, it is likely that the muscular and ligamentous structures associated with the joint will produce translational, as well as rotational, relative motion as they do in the natural joint. This additional sliding motion will almost certainly produce a greater rate of wear than that predicted by the analysis. There are two reasons for this: as the roller moves over the polyethylene surface it will (1) tend to plough through the polyethylene, and (2) subject the polyethylene to extremely high rates of loading. (The situation is equivalent to the case of a metal pin sliding on a polyethylene disc, discussed in section 2.1.2 of this chapter).

Finally, although outside the scope of this section, it is interesting to note that the requirements for a small diameter and a large angle of lap are met by polyethylene-lined hinged total knee replacements.

BIBLIOGRAPHY

Friction and Wear of Materials. (1966) E. Rabinowicz. New York and Chichester, John Wiley.
The Friction and Lubrication of Solids, Part I and Part II. (1971, 1968) F. P. Bowden and D. Tabor. Oxford, Oxford University Press.

REFERENCES

Amstutz, H. C. (1968) Polymers as bearing materials for hip replacement: a friction and wear analysis. *Journal of Biomedical Materials Research* 3, 547.
Amstutz, H. C., Lodwig, R. M., Schurman, M. D. and Hodgson, A. G. (1975) Range of motion studies for total hip replacements. *Clinical Orthopaedics and Related Research* 111, 124.
Boutin, P. (1972) Arthroplastie total de la hanche par prothèse en alumine frittée. *Revue de Chirurgie Orthopédique et Reparatrice de l'Appareil Moteur* 58, 229.
Bullough, P. G., Insall, J. N., Ranawat, C. S. and Walker, P. S. (1976) Wear and tissue reaction in failed knee arthroplasty. Communication to the British Orthopaedic Association, Spring Meeting (and in the press, *Journal of Bone and Joint Surgery*).
Charnley, J. (1970) Total hip replacement by low-friction arthroplasty. *Clinical Orthopaedics and Related Research* 72, 7.
Charnley, J. (1971) Low friction arthroplasty of the hip joint. *Journal of Bone and Joint Surgery* 53B, 149.
Charnley, J. (1974) Clinical and laboratory observations on the rate of wear of different plastic materials in the sockets of artificial hip joints. In, Biological Engineering Society Conference on 'Materials for the Use in Medicine and Biology', Churchill College, Cambridge.
Charnley, J. (1976) The wear of plastics materials in hip-joint. *Plastics and Rubber* 1, 59.

Charnley, J. and Cupic, Z. (1973) The nine and ten year results of the low-friction arthroplasty of the hip. *Clinical Orthopaedics and Related Research* **95**, 9.

Charnley, J. and Halley, D. K. (1975) Rate of wear in total hip replacement. *Clinical Orthopaedics and Related Research* **112**, 170.

Charnley, J., Kamangar, A. and Longfield, M. D. (1969) The optimum size of prosthetic heads in relation to the wear of plastic sockets in total hip replacement. *Medical and Biological Engineering* **7**, 31.

Crugnola, A. M., Radin, E. L., Rose, R. M., Paul, I. L. and Simon, S. R. (1976) Molecular weight distribution of Müller-type polyethylene components. *Transactions of the 22nd Annual Meeting of the Orthopaedic Research Society* **1**, 197.

Duff-Barclay, I. and Spillman, D. T. (1967) Total human hip joint prostheses—a laboratory study of friction and wear. *Proceedings, Institution of Mechanical Engineers* **181** (3J), 90.

Galante, J. O. and Rostoker, W. (1973) Wear in total hip prostheses. An experimental evaluation of candidate materials. *Acta Orthopaedica Scandinavica* Suppl. 145.

Gold, B. L. and Walker, P. S. (1974) Variables affecting the friction and wear of metal-on-plastic total hip joints. *Clinical Orthopaedics and Related Research* **100**, 270.

Kempson, G. E., Freeman, M. A. R. and Tuke, M. A. (1975) Engineering considerations in the design of an ankle joint. *Biomedical Engineering* **10**, 166.

Miller, D. A., Ainsworth, R. D., Dumbleton, J. H., Page, D., Miller, E. H. and Shen, Chi (1974) A comparative evaluation of the wear of ultra-high molecular weight polyethylene abraded by Ti–6Al–4V. *Wear* **28**, 207.

Paul, J. P. (1967) Forces transmitted by joints in the human body. *Proceedings, Institution of Mechanical Engineers* **181** (3J), 8.

Radin, E. L., Paul, I. L., Rose, R. M., Schiller, A. L. and Nusbaum, H. (1974) Wear and loosening of total joint replacements. *Acta Orthopaedica Belgica* **40**, 831.

Rostoker, W. and Galante, J. O. (1976) Some new studies of the wear behaviour of ultra-high molecular weight polyethylene. *Journal of Biomedical Materials Research* **10**, 303.

Scales, J. T. (1972) Some aspects of Stanmore total hip prostheses and their development. In, *Arthroplasty of the Hip*, p. 113. Ed. G. Chapchal. Stuttgart, Thieme.

Scales, J. T., Kelly, P. and Goddard, D. (1969) Friction torque studies on total joint replacements. The use of a simulator. *Annals of the Rheumatic Diseases* **28**, Suppl. 30.

Schmittgrund, G. D., Kenner, G. H. and Brown, S. D. (1973) In vivo and in vitro changes in strength of orthopaedic calcium aluminates. *Journal of Biomedical Materials Research, Symposium No. 4*, 435.

Seedhom, B. B., Dowson, D., Wright, V. and Longton, E. B. (1972) A technique for the study of geometry and contact in normal and artificial knee joints. *Wear* **20**, 189.

Simon, S. R., Paul, I. L., Rose, R. M. and Radin, E. L. (1975) 'Stiction–friction' of total hip prostheses and its relationship to loosening. *Journal of Bone and Joint Surgery* **57A**, 226.

Swanson, S. A. V., Freeman, M. A. R. and Heath, J. C. (1973) Laboratory tests on total joint replacement prostheses. *Journal of Bone and Joint Surgery* **55B**, 759.

Swikert, M. A. and Johnson, R. L. (1971) *Surface characteristics of used hip prostheses*. NASA Tech. Note TND-6153.

Ungethüm, M. and Refior, H. J. (1974) Ist Aluminiumoxidkeramik als Gleitlagerwerkstoff für Totalendoprothesen geeignet? *Archiv für Orthopädische und Unfall-Chirurgie* **79**, 97.

Walker, P. S. and Gold, B. L. (1971) The tribology (friction, lubrication and wear) of all-metal artificial hip joints. *Wear* **17,** 285.

Walker, P. S. and Gold, B. L. (1973) Comparison of the bearing performance of normal and artificial human joints. *Journal of Lubrication Technology (Trans. ASME)* July, 333.

Walker, P. S., Dowson, D., Longfield, M. D. and Wright, V. (1967) Friction and wear of artificial joint materials. *Proceedings, Institution of Mechanical Engineers* **181** (3J), 133.

Weber, B. G. (1970) Total hip replacement with rotation-endoprosthesis—trunnion-bearing prosthesis. *Clinical Orthopaedics and Related Research* **72,** 79.

Weber, B. G. and Semlitsch, I. (1972) Total hip replacement with rotation-endoprosthesis: problem of wear. In, *Arthroplasty of the Hip*, p. 71. Ed. G. Chapchal. Stuttgart, Thieme.

Weber, B. G. and Stühmer, G. (1976) Experience with trunnion bearing prosthesis with head of polyester material. In, International Symposium on Advances in Artificial Hip and Knee Joint Technology, Erlangen, W. Germany. *Engineering in Medicine*. Berlin, Springer-Verlag. In the press.

Weightman, B., Simon, S., Paul, I. L., Rose, R. and Radin, E. (1972) Lubrication mechanisms of hip joint replacement prostheses. *Journal of Lubrication Technology (Trans. ASME)* **94,** 131.

Weightman, B., Paul, I. L., Rose, R. M., Simon, S. R. and Radin, E. L. (1973) A comparative study of total hip replacement prostheses. *Journal of Biomechanics* **6,** 299.

CHAPTER FOUR

The Tissue Response to Total Joint Replacement Prostheses

1 INTRODUCTION

THE biological reactions to materials used in joint replacement procedures have been studied intensively in a few centres in recent years. While some studies have been directed towards an understanding of the nature of the normal bond between the implant and bone, others have been directed primarily towards the pathogenesis of loosening of prostheses especially in those cases in which the technique of implantation appears to have been satisfactory, in which there is no history of injury, and in which there is no evidence by conventional criteria of the presence of infection. The very good results which are generally observed in the period immediately following total joint replacement are, regrettably, no guarantee of permanent success in the long term, since, even if a prosthesis is firmly fixed in place for a short or long period after implantation, various factors can eventually lead to loosening at a later date. Clearly, at the forefront of any discussion of the causes of prosthetic loosening must be a consideration of the possible sequelae of the interaction between the body tissues and the components of the implant and their wear and corrosion products. Any consideration of the biological reaction to the implant materials may be relevant not only to loosening, but also to the causation of pain, infection, hypersensitivity to implant materials, and neoplasia.

In this chapter, current knowledge will be reviewed with particular regard to (1) the reaction of the bone to the implant, (2) the reactions of the tissues to wear products, and (3) the role of these reactions in the causation of the complications of total joint replacement.

2 THE REACTION OF BONE TO AN IMPLANT

2.1 The Morphology of the Normal Bone–Cement Interface

With most of the total joint endoprostheses in use at the present time, one or both of the prosthetic components are fixed into bone using one of the self-curing acrylic cements. When considering the nature of the 'implant bed' one is primarily concerned, therefore, with the interaction between bone and bone marrow tissues on the one hand and the acrylic cement bonding the endoprosthesis in place on the other. Although there should be (in theory at least) little or no contact between the metallic or plastic components of the endoprosthesis and bone or marrow tissues as far as the normal implant bed is concerned, evidence will be cited later to show that the metallic or plastic components of prostheses may play a key role in the breakdown of the bond between acrylic cement and bone in cases of late loosening.

There is general agreement regarding the early and late histopathological changes in the bone adjoining acrylic cement bonding prostheses in place in man. These have been studied and described by Charnley (1970), Willert and his colleagues (Willert and Puls 1972; Willert 1973; Willert et al. 1974), and by Vernon-Roberts and Freeman (1976). In summary, it may be considered that the tissue reaction after implantation passes through three phases: (1) an initial phase which lasts from the time of implantation to about three weeks after operation; (2) a reparative phase beginning during about the fourth week after operation and lasting for up to two years; and (3) a stabilisation phase which begins six months to two years after operation. While this division of the tissue reaction in the implant bed into these three phases aids the understanding of the underlying pathological processes, it must be borne in mind that there are wide variations in the duration of these phases in individual cases.

In the *initial phase*, the outer surface of the cement has uniform contact with surrounding body tissues such that where protruding plugs of cement are present they fit into hollows having a similar shape in the tissues. There is no gross movement between the cement and the bone irrespective of whether the outer surface of the cement is relatively smooth or has a nodular surface when examined macroscopically. However, cement surfaces having multiple protruding plugs of cement are more difficult to remove from the bone bed (Vernon-Roberts and Freeman 1976), and this suggests that these 'rough-surfaced' implants are more firmly bonded into the bone than 'smooth-surfaced' implants, at least in the initial stage.

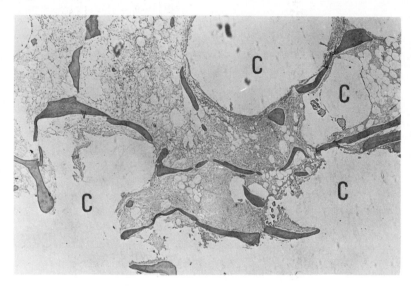

Figure 4.1.
Implant bed 10 days after implantation. The trabecular bone and bone marrow adjoining the cement (C) is all dead. Spaces in the tissues are occupied by cement masses separate from the cement bonding the prosthesis in place. Haematoxylin–eosin × 15.

Histological examination of the implant bed in the initial stage always reveals a zone of dead bone and bone marrow extending up to 5 mm from the cement surface (Fig. 4.1). Less frequently, larger areas of necrosis of cancellous and of compact cortical bone may also be present. The constant presence of a zone of necrotic bone and bone marrow immediately surrounding the cement suggests that local tissue death results from reaming or cutting the bone, from the heat produced during polymerisation of monomeric methyl methacrylate, from the toxic effects of released monomer, or from a combination of these factors (see section 2.2.1 of this chapter); the death of larger areas of cancellous bone and of cortical bone not in close contact with cement cannot easily be ascribed to these factors and clearly must be the result of an interruption of the vascular supply to the involved areas during the surgical procedure of implantation (Fig. 4.2). At the junction between dead and living bone there are vascular dilatation, an exudation of inflammatory cells, proliferation of blood vessels, and the appearance of fibroblasts, osteoclasts and osteoblasts; these findings are identical with the initial reaction of the living vascularised tissues around any piece of infarcted bone. Thus, during the initial phase, the cement bonding the prosthesis into the implant bed is in contact only with dead bone and dead bone marrow to which the adjacent living tissues react in the usual fashion.

An additional constant microscopic finding in the dead tissue in the implant bed is the presence of variable amounts of cement separate from the main cement mass; these separate pieces of cement may occasionally be composed of aggregates large enough to be seen easily with the naked eye, but separate discrete 'acrylic pearls' (spheres of cement up to 80 μm in diameter) are always present lying singly or aggregated together.

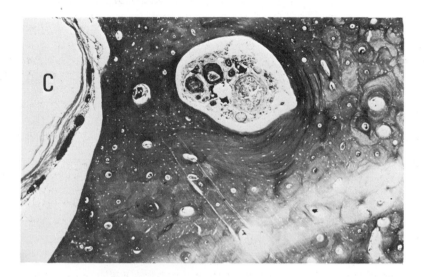

Figure 4.2.
(a) Cortical bone separated from cement (C) by a layer of fibrous tissue one year after implantation. The cortical bone exhibits death of bone around a vascular channel. Haematoxylin–eosin × 50. (b) Higher magnification of vascular channel shown in (a). Shows dead original blood vessels and ingrowth of new artery (arrow). × 120.

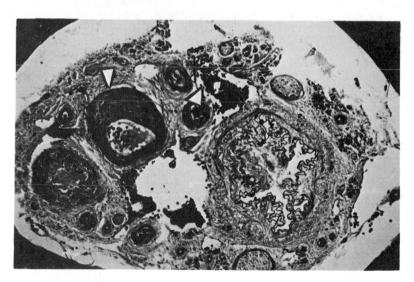

In the *reparative phase* the dead tissues are progressively invaded by living vascular granulation tissue bringing with it scavenger cells which remove dead bone and bone marrow, and connective tissue cells which lay down fibrous tissue and new bone. The dead bone is removed by the activity of osteoclasts. However, some of the dead trabeculae of cancellous bone gain a covering of new living bone before all of the dead bone has been removed, and these 'composite trabeculae', having a core of dead bone covered by living bone, may persist for several years in the tissues close to the surface of the main cement mass (Fig. 4.3). In some cases, at the junction of dead and living bone there is marked buttressing of dead bone by the surface accretion of nodular masses of new living bone (Fig. 4.4). This seems to be a temporary phenomenon occurring soon after implantation, and it would appear that these nodular buttresses are eventually remodelled to form normal trabeculae.

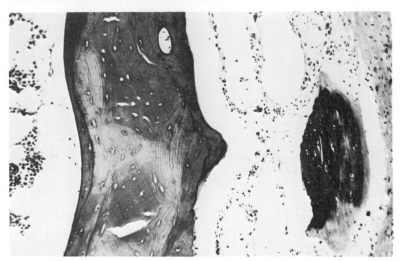

Figure 4.3.
Implant bed two years after implantation. Fibrous tissue separating cement from bone is at right of micrograph. Shows 'composite' trabecula having central core of dead bone (note empty osteocyte lacunae) surrounded by living bone. Haematoxylin–eosin × 120.

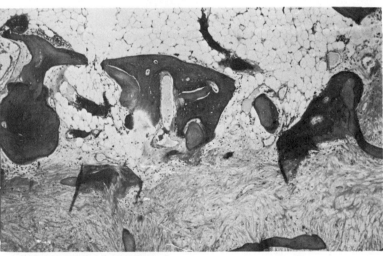

Figure 4.4.
Implant bed one year after implantation. The bone and bone marrow in the upper half of the micrograph is dead. Shows buttressing of dead trabeculae by surface apposition of new bone at the junction of living and dead tissue. Haematoxylin–eosin × 50.

At the junction between the main cement mass and the revascularised implant bed, the cement is separated from the living tissues by at least an acellular layer which may be exceedingly thin and delicate (Fig. 4.5) and has the appearance of fibrin. In addition to this inner acellular fibrin-like layer in contact with the cement, there is usually an outer layer of collagenised fibrous tissue up to 1 mm thick (Fig. 4.6). It has been reported that this fibrous tissue may undergo metaplasia to fibrocartilage (Charnley 1970). On rare occasions, parts of the surface abutting on to the cement are lined by numerous foreign-body giant cells (Fig. 4.7a) which may be seen to contain intracellular small spherules having the appearances of prepolymerised methyl methacrylate (Fig. 4.7b).

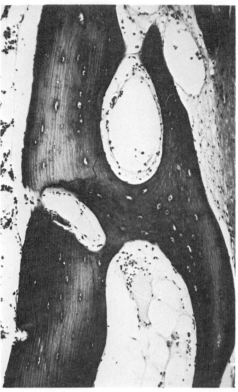
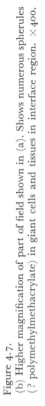

Figure 4.5.
Implant bed one year after implantation. Cement (C) is separated from the bone by a thin acellular layer. Haematoxylin–eosin × 120.

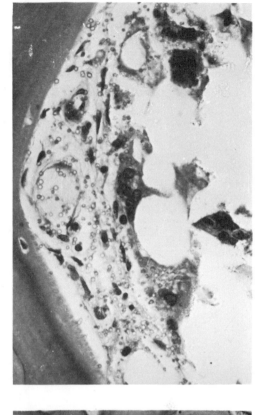

Figure 4.6.
Implant bed one year after implantation. Bone is separated from cement by the layer of heavily collagenised fibrous tissue seen at the bottom of the micrograph. Haematoxylin–eosin × 120.

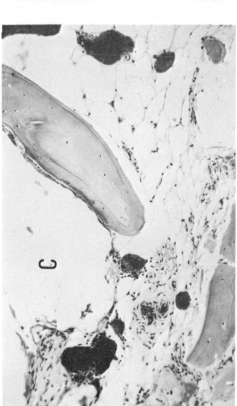
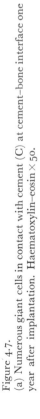

Figure 4.7.
(a) Numerous giant cells in contact with cement (C) at cement-bone interface one year after implantation. Haematoxylin–eosin × 50.

Figure 4.7.
(b) Higher magnification of part of field shown in (a). Shows numerous spherules (? polymethylmethacrylate) in giant cells and tissues in interface region. × 400.

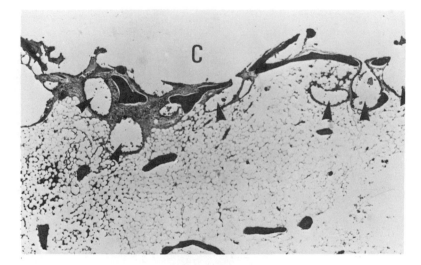

Figure 4.8.
Implant bed 10 months after implantation. Shows spaces (arrows) occupied by spheres of cement, some of which are extensions of the main cement mass (C). Haematoxylin–eosin × 15.

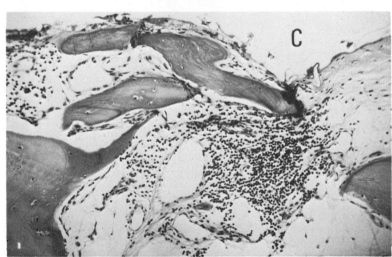

Figure 4.9.
Perivascular lymphocytic infiltration in soft tissue adjacent to cement (C) one year after implantation. Haematoxylin–eosin × 120.

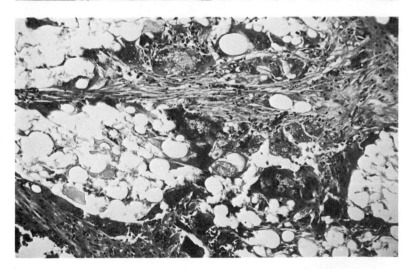

Figure 4.10.
Large numbers of multinucleate giant cells containing acrylic cement fragments and removing necrotic fatty marrow in implant bed surrounding a painful prosthesis one year after implantation. Haematoxylin–eosin × 120.

In the tissues within approximately 5 mm of the main cement mass (as distinct from at the interface itself), separate pieces of cement and single and aggregated acrylic pearls become surrounded by multinucleate giant cells which frequently form a syncytium having few visible cell boundaries (Fig. 4.8, and see Fig. 4.18). In this area there is also very active bone formation and remodelling, fibrous tissue formation, perivascular lymphocytic infiltrates (Fig. 4.9), occasional hyaline cartilage formation, and foamy macrophages and multinucleate giant cells removing necrotic marrow tissue and containing acrylic cement (Fig. 4.10). Haemopoietic marrow may make its appearance very close to the cement surface (Fig. 4.11). Small foci of dead bone marrow tissue sometimes persist without further evidence of attempts at their repair, but these do not appear to be associated with early or late loosening of the implant.

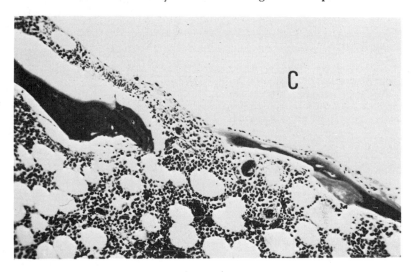

Figure 4.11.
Haemopoietic marrow lying close to cement (C) surface two years after implantation. Haematoxylin–eosin × 120.

The active repair process proceeds until all, or almost all, of the dead tissues have been replaced by living bone and living soft connective tissues. After this has been achieved, a stable state is eventually established between the implant and its bed. The implant may therefore be considered to be healed into place during the *stabilisation phase* which begins one or two years after operation (Willert 1973). Although as histologically defined this phase rarely starts in less than one year after implantation, bone blood flow as measured by the uptake of bone-seeking isotopes appears to return to normal by six months (Feith et al. 1976).

The 'permanent' implant bed is composed of a thin layer of acellular fibrin-like tissue in immediate contact with the main cement mass, with or without an outer layer of collagenised fibrous tissue up to 1.5 mm thick (Fig. 4.12). The separate pieces of cement and acrylic pearls persist, are surrounded by a thin syncytium of giant cells and may become embedded in fibrous tissue. Other multinucleate giant cells may contain particles of cement. Inflammatory cells are sparse although scattered foci of perivascular lymphocytes may be present close to the main cement mass. The granulation tissue which occupied the marrow spaces during the reparative phase is replaced by normal fatty and haemopoietic marrow tissue, and the dead bone and woven repair bone of that phase is replaced by mature lamellar trabecular bone. While many of the new trabeculae are orientated perpendicular to the surface of the main cement mass, those nearest the cement frequently become orientated parallel to the cement surface (Fig. 4.13).

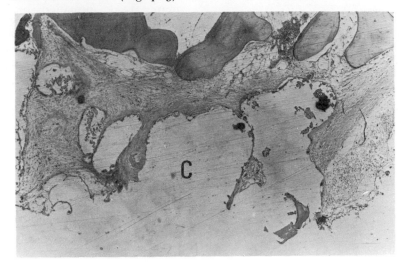

Figure 4.12.
Implant bed two years after implantation. Shows cement (C) separated from bone by a thick layer of fibrous tissue containing some isolated spheres of cement. (Scratch marks are in fact score marks made by the knife going across the section.) Haematoxylin–eosin × 30.

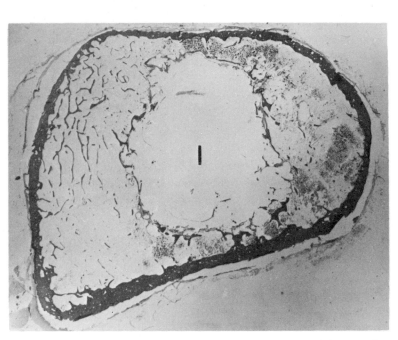

Figure 4.13.
Section through shaft of femur of patient who died two years after implantation. The implant (I) was stable. The trabeculae nearest the cement are orientated parallel to the cement surface. The remainder of the cancellous bone is porotic. The cortex is united to the trabeculae around the implant by a few radially orientated trabeculae. Haematoxylin–eosin × 4.

In some cases of intramedullary stem fixation, many of the trabeculae situated between the inner cortex near the bone end and the trabeculae closely encircling the cement disappear to leave the inner and outer bone connected only by a few radially orientated trabeculae (Fig. 4.13). This reduction in the amount of cancellous bone (i.e. porosis or bone wasting) presumably occurs because the bone is no longer required to provide a supporting function (see Chapter 2, section 3.2), a process similar to disuse-osteoporosis from other causes.

2.2 The Cause of Fibrous Tissue Formation at the Bone–Cement Interface

Since in cemented prostheses the cement is initially in direct contact with dead bone and since in the stabilisation phase it is usually separated from living bone by fibrous tissue, it must follow that in the reparative phase some dead bone undergoes fibrous replacement. The following two questions must therefore be asked when considering the cause of fibrous tissue formation around a cemented implant: (1) why does the bone die? and (2) why is it partly replaced by fibrous tissue instead of by living bone?

2.2.1 THE CAUSE OF BONE DEATH

The cause of the death of bone at the bone–cement interface is uncertain but three factors have been implicated: (1) the trauma and heat generated by cutting and reaming the bone, (2) the heat generated by the polymerisation of polymethylmethacrylate (PMMA), and (3) leakage of monomer from the cement before it polymerises. Perhaps all of these factors are responsible to an extent which varies from case to case.

That atraumatic handling of the bone is important has been demonstrated by Linder and Lundskog (1975) who claimed to show that if the operative technique was sufficiently gentle, direct contact could be achieved and maintained between living cortical bone and a metallic implant. So close can this contact be that considerable forces may be required to extract even smooth-surfaced implants.

Polymethylmethacrylate generates significant heat when it polymerises so that thermal necrosis of bone is clearly a possibility. Doubt, however, has been cast on the extent to which this occurs in practice (Jefferiss, Lee and Ling 1975) since flowing blood and metallic implants may both act, in different ways, as effective heat sinks to reduce the surface temperature of the cement mass at operation. Temperatures reached during the implantation with cement of a Thompson femoral head prosthesis into a cadaveric femur heated to 37°C were measured by Ohnsorge and Goebel (1970). The highest temperature of the bone–cement interface was in the greater trochanter, and reached 72°C when the prosthesis was initially at 25°C, but only 53°C when the prosthesis had previously been cooled to 0°C; the authors regard this difference as significant since protein denatures at 56°C. Biehl, Harms and Hanser (1974) made similar measurements at the bone–cement interface within the greater trochanter and elsewhere, but *in vivo*. No temperature higher than 46°C was recorded. With a prosthesis cooled to 0°C, all the interfacial temperatures were reduced by about 5°C. At both the tibial and femoral bone–cement interfaces of an unspecified knee prosthesis, maximum temperatures between 53 and 65°C were recorded. The authors attribute the difference between the knee and hip temperatures to the reduced heat transfer from the bone consequent on the haemostasis enforced during knee replacement under a tourniquet. The difference between their measurements on the hip *in vivo* and those of Ohnsorge and Goebel *in vitro* were similarly explained by the presence and absence respectively of blood flow. Labitzke and Paulus (1974) made similar measurements in the hip, and obtained maximum interfacial temperatures of 41–49°C in the acetabulum.

The prostheses were of the Müller type, having high density poly-ethylene cups and, as the authors remark, the considerably lower thermal conductivity of this material would be expected to lead to higher interfacial temperatures than with metallic components. These authors quote unpublished work showing that the coagulation temperature of bone collagen is at least 70°C, and conclude that the danger of thermal damage to the matrix in clinical practice is remote. Damage to the cells is, of course, more likely.

Monomeric methyl methacrylate is toxic and diffuses from the cement mass before full polymerisation. That it may cause toxic necrosis of the adjacent bone is therefore reasonable (Charnley 1970) but as yet unproven. None of the modern implantable alloys nor polymerised acrylic cement itself causes bone death (Linder and Lundskog 1975).

Thus of the three factors which might be responsible for the initial death of bone at the bone–cement interface, trauma seems to be the most likely and factors specific to PMMA cement the least likely.

2.2.2 THE CAUSE OF FIBROUS REPLACEMENT OF DEAD BONE

Dead cancellous bone is revascularised and converted to intact living cancellous tissue by the ingrowth of granulation tissue, the deposition of living appositional woven bone upon the dead trabecula and finally the modelling of these 'composite' trabecula to form normal living bone. This process requires an intact scaffold of dead cancellous bone through which granulation tissue can advance and upon which living bone can be laid down. If the dead bone fractures (so presumably permitting movement between the fracture surfaces at each load application) the area in question generally undergoes fibrous rather than bony replacement. This suggests that the fundamental event making for fibrous replacement of the dead bone at the cement interface in man is fracture of the dead cancellous tissue.

Dead bone tested in the laboratory is fatigue-prone (Swanson, Freeman and Day 1971). Dead bone is not turned over as is living bone, so its matrix will steadily accumulate load cycles. Thus it seems possible that the dead cancellous bone adjacent to the cement mass may eventually suffer fatigue fracture in the face of the repetitive loads applied in everyday life. The longer the period for which the bone is loaded, the more likely this is to occur.

Clearly the length of time which it takes for the dead bone to be revascularised, removed, and then replaced by new living bone is largely determined by the extent of the initial bone death: when there has been extensive bone death, the cement must remain anchored to dead bone for a longer period than if bone death were minimal. Thus it seems likely that the more extensive is the initial infarct, the greater is the likelihood of eventual fatigue fracture and hence of fibrous replacement.

A second factor which may be responsible for fracture derives from recent animal studies which indicate that the bone of the experimentally infarcted femoral head is weaker in the face of statically applied loads than is the bone of the normal femoral head (Szepesi and Kapitany 1974; Szepezi, Kapitany and Csorba 1974).

Thus dead, repetitively loaded cancellous bone may undergo fibrous replacement because it fractures and it may fracture because it suffers fatigue failure or because its static mechanical properties are impaired.

2.3 Direct Contact between Prostheses and Living Bone

The first implants used for joint replacement were fixed to the skeleton simply as push fits and therefore must initially have made direct contact with bone. Clinical experience, however, showed that devices attached to the skeleton in this way (such as the Thompson prosthesis) tended to loosen. Therefore two lines of development took place. On the one hand the stem of the prosthesis was fenestrated in the hope of inducing bone to grow into the implant and lock it to the skeleton (an example of such a device was the Moore prosthesis). On the other hand, total contact and interlocking between the implant and the skeleton were achieved by the use of polymethylmethacrylate. Unfortunately, the first attempts to produce stabilisation of a prosthesis in the skeleton by bone growth and interlocking were not regularly successful, whilst (fortunately) the use of acrylic cement was attended with a very high incidence of clinical success. Although clinical success is usual with the use of acrylic cement, it is not invariable: some prostheses loosen, even as late as six years after implantation. This subject is considered in more detail in section 4.1 of this chapter and section 3 of Chapter 5; here it suffices to say that the view has gained ground that late loosening of the implant may be related to the presence of a fibrous tissue layer between the living bone and the cement. Once again, therefore, attempts are being made to implant prostheses in such a way that living bone is in direct, permanent contact with large areas of the surface of the implant and, if possible, to induce bone to grow into the implant itself so as to lock it in place.

In seeking direct contact between the implant and living bone rather than between the implant and fibrous tissue, orthopaedic surgeons have perhaps been influenced by their experience with fracture union and ankylosis. In these situations, a direct bone bridge across the fusion site is attended by permanent stability, the absence of recurrent deformation, and the absence of pain. In contrast, the presence of fibrous tissue at the fusion site may be accompanied by pain and progressive recurrent deformity which, in the context of joint replacement, is the equivalent of loosening.

Although the analogy with fracture union is attractive, it remains an analogy and not a statement of demonstrated fact. Clearly, if the zone of fibrous replacement in a cemented prosthesis is large in relation to the bony prominences upon which interlock depends, loosening is likely. In practice, however, it is by no means certain that this is a common cause of loosening and if it occurs less frequently than bone fails to grow into an implant, the clinical incidence of loosening with cemented prostheses should be lower than that associated with implants dependent on bone ingrowth.

To achieve permanent, direct contact between living bone and the material of an implant two broad requirements must be met: firstly, techniques must be available by which living bone can be brought into close proximity to the surface of an implant at the time of operation and then maintained there by a suitable postoperative regime; and secondly, implant materials must be selected which will encourage bone to grow up to the surface of, and into pores in, the implant.

The clinical experience obtained with cemented implants has shown that if a prosthesis is to remain symptomless over a period of years, the stresses on the interface must be low enough to avoid fatigue failure of the involved bone (that is to say, the area of contact must be high) and little or no movement must occur between the implant and the skeleton. These two objectives can be achieved at the time of operation with cement since the dead space between the irregular surface of the bone and the regular surface of the prosthesis can be filled with cement which moulds itself to the two surfaces as it polymerises. If comparable contact is to be achieved without the use of cement, very precise surgical techniques will have to be achieved since the capacity of bone to grow beyond its confines to fill a 'dead space' is limited: perhaps gaps of 2 mm represent the practical limit. Obviously, if there is to be no movement between the prosthesis and the skeleton in the first instance, an exact fit will have to be obtained at least in certain mechanically crucial parts of the implant surface, whilst if the stresses are not to be unacceptably high on these contacting areas, the percentage of the implant surface forming an exact fit with the skeleton will have to be high. Thus to achieve permanent contact with living bone it would appear that prostheses will have to be implanted in such a way that they make perfect contact with the skeleton over much of their surface, doing so in particular in those areas upon which the initial fixation depends, and that in areas in which imperfect contact is made the bone will have to be separated by not more than about 2 mm from the implant. In practice this will be at best difficult, at worst impossible. It seems unlikely, for example, that it will prove possible regularly to achieve this accuracy of contact over the surface of an intramedullary stem, whilst for 'resurfacing' prostheses the disease process itself may render this objective difficult to attain: both rheumatoid arthritis and osteoarthrosis are characterised by the development of lesions ('cysts') within the juxta-articular skeleton which would have to be filled in some way by the implant itself if cement were not to be employed.

Assuming that on the gross scale the appropriate bony surfaces could be fashioned, it would further be necessary either to cut the bone in such a way that it was not killed during the course of preparation, or to reduce the loads applied to the replaced joint for a sufficient period of time to allow the replacement of any dead bone with living bone. That cortical bone can be cut in such a way as to leave living bone in contact with an implant has been claimed by Linder and Lundskog (1975) but the necessary techniques may be difficult to achieve in routine surgical practice. To prepare cancellous bone in this way seems likely to be even more difficult, if not impossible. Nevertheless, it has recently been demonstrated (Brånemark et al. 1975) that it is possible to transmit load through titanium screws inserted into the human mandible provided (1) that the insertion technique is sufficiently gentle, and (2) that the implants are not loaded for an initial period after their insertion during which the bone in the implant bed matures. In the clinical context of joint replacement, the problem arises that for patients whose joints need replacement, weight relief for several months postoperatively is frequently impossible. (Indeed, if weight-relief could be practised routinely with cemented prostheses, it might well be that fibrous tissue would be absent from their interfaces.)

If it is thought necessary to lock the prosthesis into living bone in such a way that it can resist loads applied from any direction, the ingrowth of bone into the implant will have to be achieved (see Chapter 5, section 3.7).In the limit an implant fixed in any other way (for example, by being formed as a screw) could always be loosened by reversing the forces required for its insertion. Bone can certainly be induced to grow into an implant (see section 2.3.2 of this chapter) but only if movement between the implant and the skeleton is prevented, at least for the first three to six months. If movement is permitted, a fibrous envelope develops round the prosthesis (see, for example, Lundskog 1972; Cameron, Pilliar and MacNab 1973; Uhtoff 1973; Linder and Lundskog 1975). A period of immobilisation is necessary because the ingrowth of bone is preceded by the ingrowth of blood vessels in a loose connective tissue stroma. If the implant is allowed to slide over the bony skeleton by even a millimetre or two, this tissue is damaged and the ingrowth of bone prevented.

To achieve this degree of implant immobilisation, both a very precise surgical technique and a reduction in the loads applied to the joint seem likely to be needed. The practical difficulties in the way of achieving both these objectives have already been referred to. Nevertheless, bone ingrowth has been reported in porous intramedullary prosthetic stems and porous staples loaded immediately after implantation in dogs and rabbits (Cameron, MacNab and Pilliar 1972; Homsy et al. 1972; Lembert, Galante and Rostoker 1972) so that the requisite degree of immobilisation is certainly attainable.

A second prerequisite for bone ingrowth is that the indentations in the implant into which bone is to grow must be above a certain minimum size. This topic has been studied by Klawitter and Hulbert (1971), Lembert, Galante and Rostoker (1972), Howe, Svare and Tock (1975) and others in the context of porous surface. Regardless of the material, pore sizes greater than about 100 μm (0·1 mm) have produced histological evidence of ingrowth, strengths suggesting significant ingrowth, or both. This generalisation can be refined a little. Klawitter and Hulbert (1971) found in calcium aluminate that fibrous tissue grew into pores 5–15 μm in diameter, osteoid tissue into pores 40–100 μm, and bone into pores 100 μm or greater in diameter; Lembert, Galante and Rostoker (1972) found that variations of pore size in the range of 190–390 μm gave no significant variation in the shear strength six weeks after implantation in dogs; Welsh, Pilliar and MacNab (1971) obtained shear strengths with porous Co–Cr–Mo alloy suggesting considerable bone ingrowth, with pores of a size not stated by the authors but apparently, from scanning electron micrographs, in the range 10–20 μm; and Nilles, Coletti and Wilson (1973) found that pyrolytic carbon with a pore size in the range 3–10 μm gave shear strengths similar to those obtained with solid-surfaced stainless steel; Howe, Svare and Tock (1975) found, within the range of 275–670 μm, the greatest filling of a single pore when this had a diameter of 420 μm.

Thus it seems that in any material into which bone will grow, a pore size of 100 μm or greater will ensure adequate ingrowth; smaller pores may allow ingrowth, but there seems no reason to prefer them.

The maximum extent to which human bone will grow into a dead space from a cut surface of bone is not known, but it would appear to be of the order of 1–2 mm. Gaps larger than this may be bridged at fracture surfaces but there the biological environment is somewhat different. If the maximum capacity for outgrowth for practical purposes were to be regarded as being 1 mm, it would seem pointless to have indentations in a prosthetic surface larger than this, since to do so would only increase the chance of filling the recess partly with bone and partly with fibrous tissue.

Therefore it would appear that when it is hoped to encourage bone growth into implant surfaces, (1) the whole of the surface which contacts bone should be serrated or porous, and (2) the recesses or pores in the prosthesis should be between 0.1 and 1 mm in diameter and depth, with a possible optimum at 0.5 mm.

At the present time, attempts are being made in a number of centres to fix total joint prostheses in man without the use of cement by making use of the principles of surgical accuracy, postoperative weight-relief and suitably porous or serrated prosthetic surfaces. Although encouraging clinical results have been reported, it would be premature to comment on them here since the periods of follow-up are as yet short and the supporting histological data scanty.

The maximum distance over which reliable bone outgrowth can be expected (1–2 mm) is about equal to the depth of surface depressions which have been found to have been filled by a fibrous tissue layer after one year of weight-bearing in the dog (Biehl, Harms and Mäusle 1975). This raises the possibilities that the presence or absence of repeated loads is the critical factor, and that an implant with surface porosities about 1 mm in linear dimensions will provoke the same reactions as one with grooves about 1 mm deep. If this is so, longer clinical experience may show that with either porous or grooved surfaces the repeated application of load brings about the fibrous replacement of bone which has formed during an initial phase of restricted loading.

2.3.2 THE INFLUENCE OF THE MATERIAL OF THE IMPLANT UPON ITS PERMANENT CONTACT WITH LIVING BONE

Although some implant materials are said to be particularly appropriate for use in this context because they are biologically more inert (for example, ceramic corrodes less than does cobalt–chromium alloy), it would appear that all of the materials in current clinical use and several other experimental materials will permit living bone to exist in immediate contact with them.

Bone ingrowth has been observed in sintered calcium aluminate (Klawitter and Hulbert 1971; Nilles, Coletti and Wilson 1973), sintered alumina (Hulbert et al. 1974), ceramic made from alumina, silica, calcium carbonate and magnesium carbonate (Welsh, Pilliar and MacNab 1971), ceramic containing 96 per cent alumina with silica, magnesium oxide and traces of other metallic oxides (Lyng et al. 1973), sintered titanium wire (Galante et al. 1971; Lembert, Galante and Rostoker 1972), sintered Co–Cr–Mo alloy balls (Cameron, Pilliar and MacNab 1973), sintered stainless steel (Nilles, Coletti and Wilson 1973), polytetrafluorethylene and pyrolytic graphite (Homsy et al. 1972), polytetrafluorethylene (Howe, Svare and Tock 1975), pyrolytic graphite (Nilles, Coletti and Wilson 1973) and polyethylene (Klawitter et al. 1976; Sauer et al. 1976).

Stainless steel and Co–Cr–Mo alloy have been used in orthopaedic implants for many years and are known to produce very few if any significant adverse reactions. Thus their use in this context is attractive. On the other hand, as some of the authors cited above have remarked, a porous-surfaced metal implant presents a total surface area many orders of magnitude larger than an equivalent smooth-surfaced implant, and the possibility of unacceptably increased reaction is thereby introduced. Nevertheless, porous metal implants are now being considered for clinical use, especially in North America. A possible solution to the potential problem of increased surface reactivity was suggested by Nilles, Coletti and Wilson (1973) who pointed out that the sintering of stainless steel or titanium produced an oxide film on the entire surface of the porous metal mass and that this could be expected to make the implant more inert. This would also be true of the titanium tested by Galante and co-workers. However, since these two materials owe their corrosion resistance to naturally formed oxide films, the effect of sintering is to produce not a difference of kind but one of degree, by giving (unless the sintering is performed in an inert atmosphere) a thicker and perhaps stronger oxide film.

Ceramics, being metallic oxides, would be expected to be chemically and hence biologically more inert than pure metals and alloys. Interest in ceramics as implant materials is particularly strong in Continental Europe where a number of ceramic prostheses have been used clinically (cf. Boutin 1974; Mittelmeier 1975). In partial support of the belief that direct contact might readily be achieved between living bone and ceramic, Hulbert et al. (1974) observed the presence of an osteoid seam 10–50 μm thick between bone and calcium aluminate (a ceramic) but not between bone and aluminium oxide (another ceramic). Direct bone contact was also observed by Lyng et al. (1973) with their 96 per cent alumina ceramic. In contrast, other workers have reported that ceramic implants are separated from bone by a zone of fibrous tissue in exactly the same way as are metals (Geduldig et al. 1975). It is too early yet to say whether or not ceramic materials have particular advantages in this respect but the impression emerges that they have not (Willert, personal communication 1976).

2.3.3 SUMMARY

Three factors have been shown to be important if living bone is to be in permanent contact with an implant. Firstly, the preparation of the bone surface must be as atraumatic as possible and must shape the bone to be an exact fit for the prosthesis. Secondly, the prosthesis must be immobilised on the bone for the first three to six months after implantation, a requirement which makes weight-bearing on the limb undesirable. Finally the implant must be biologically inert, a requirement which in the light of present knowledge appears to be equally well met by several metals, metal oxides (ceramics) and polymers. If bone is to grow into (as against merely up to) an implant, the surface of the prosthesis must be serrated or porous and the pores or serrations should be between 0·1 and 1·0 mm in diameter. Although these four factors have been shown to be important and relevant, the literature contains few studies in which they have been investigated individually. Thus at present their relative importance has not been finally established.

3 THE 'NORMAL' TISSUE RESPONSE TO WEAR DEBRIS AND SOLUTES

Some degree of wear of the bearing surfaces of total joint replacement endoprostheses is inevitable, and particulate products of wear may thus be formed from the bearing surfaces of both metal and plastic components. The rates and mechanisms of wear in different types of prostheses are discussed in Chapter 3.

Corrosion of metal components and of metallic wear particles leads to the formation of soluble and insoluble compounds. Wear is not essential for the release of metal into the tissues since, in studies of metal levels in the tissues surrounding implanted cobalt–chromium and stainless steel cylinders, the constituent metals were detected in the tissues four to six months after implantation (Ferguson, Laing and Hodge 1960). However, the enormously larger surface area presented by wear particles would be expected to result in the solution of much larger amounts of metal by the corrosion of wear particles than by the corrosion of the original bearing surface, a theoretical expectation which has been demonstrated in the case of cobalt–chromium wear particles from which metal rapidly dissolves in horse serum (Swanson, Freeman and Heath 1973). Evidence for the release of metals from prostheses in man was obtained by Coleman, Herrington and Scales (1973) who found that in nine patients with prostheses composed of cobalt–chromium articulating with cobalt–chromium both blood and urinary cobalt and chromium levels were persistently elevated, whereas in three patients with prostheses composed of cobalt–chromium articulating against high molecular weight polyethylene they were unable to detect a significant elevation of blood and urinary cobalt and chromium levels. Owen, Meachim and Williams (1976) reported no significant increase in the chromium content of hair from 62 patients with hip prostheses in which stainless steel articulated against polyethylene, compared with 51 control subjects. These clinical observations are in agreement with the findings of Swanson, Freeman and Heath (1973), who used laboratory simulators to show that prostheses in which both components were composed of cobalt–chromium released both cobalt and chromium into the solution bathing the bearing surfaces during the test, whereas prostheses in which cobalt–chromium or stainless steel articulated against high density polyethylene did not release detectable amount of metal under similar laboratory conditions.

Thus, in all patients in whom prostheses having bearing surfaces have been implanted, constituents of the implant materials are being constantly liberated by wear and corrosion into the tissues surrounding the prosthesis, whence they may be mobilised to other parts of the body. It is therefore of fundamental importance that the nature of the tissue reactions to the metallic and plastic debris from prostheses should be understood.

3.1 The Morphology of the Soft Tissue Reactions to Particles Containing Metal and to Particles of Polyethylene and Other Non-metallics

The histological response of the connective tissues of the joint cavity to the products of wear and corrosion of prostheses have been the subject of a number of recent studies which are in general agreement (Semlitsch, Vogel and Willert 1972; Willert 1973; Evans et al. 1974; Willert and Semlitsch 1974; Winter 1974; Vernon-Roberts and Freeman 1976). The findings summarised here are based upon the published work of Willert and his colleagues, and upon the studies of Vernon-Roberts and Freeman who have carried out detailed combined morphological and analytical studies of the tissues obtained at operation or post-mortem from around nearly 100 prostheses.

After the implantation of an all-cobalt–chromium or a metal–polyethylene prosthesis, a new fibrous connective tissue capsule is formed around the articulation if the original articular capsule has been excised. Whether the articulation is surrounded by the original capsule or a new capsule, the general structure of the lining soon resembles synovial membrane and may continue to do so for a long period. However, in most cases, the lining tissues eventually undergo characteristic morphological changes associated with the presence of foreign material. When these changes are well developed, the most striking feature is the presence of numerous macrophages and multinucleate giant cells (Fig. 4.14). These may be arranged in extensive confluent sheets, nodules separated by thick or thin bands of fibrous tissue, or as small clusters of cells interspersed in dense fibrous tissue. Frequently, lymphocytes and plasma cells are present among the macrophages, particularly in the regions around small blood vessels; occasional neutrophil and eosinophil polymorphs may also be observed but they are not a constant or marked feature of the cellular response.

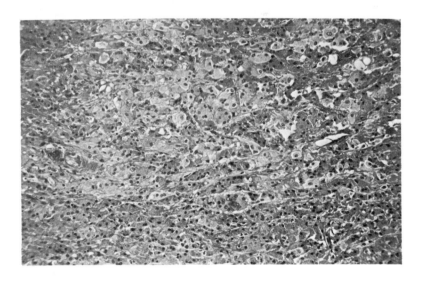

Figure 4.14.
Sheet of macrophages and giant cells in articular tissues 15 months after implantation of a cobalt–chrome against high density polyethylene knee prosthesis which became painful. Haematoxylin–eosin × 120.

Table 4.1 Light Microscopic Appearances of Intracellular Foreign Material in Tissues Adjacent to Joint Prostheses

Prosthesis material	Type of tissue reaction				Morphology of intracellular material	Maximum dimensions of particles	Birefringence
	Macrophages	Giant cells	Necrosis	Fibrosis			
Metal (cobalt–chromium or stainless steel)	++++	++	++++	++	Black granules, rods and needles	0·1–3·0 μm	Strong: granules, rods and needles
Polyethylene	+++	++++	±	++++	Colourless	0·5–50 μm	Strong: diffuse intracellular mottling, spears, splinters, sheets
Polymethyl-methacrylate	++	++++	—	+	Empty spaces* in form of spheres, ovoids and splinters	0·5–80 μm	Very weak

* Readily soluble in solvents used in routine processing.

Figure 4.15.
(a) Numerous small black metallic particles in macrophages and giant cells in articular tissues one year after implantation of an all-cobalt–chronium knee prosthesis which became persistently painful. Haematoxylin–eosin × 400. (b) Same field as (a), viewed between crossed polars. Shows strong birefringence of the intracellular crystalline particles. (The dust particles are in fact in the mounting medium.)

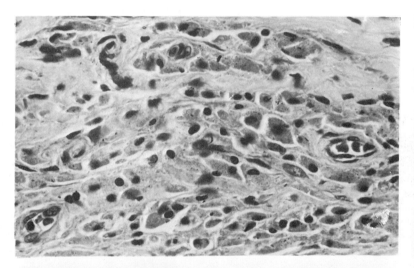

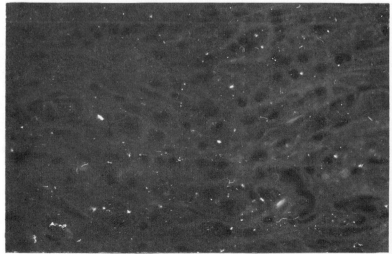

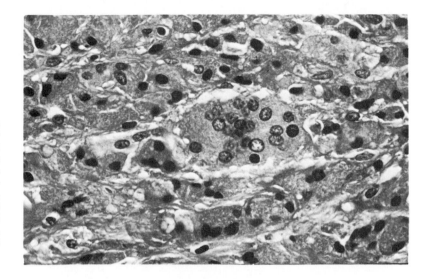

Figure 4.16.
(a) Macrophage and giant cell reaction in articular tissues 15 months after implantation of a cobalt–chromium against high density polyethylene knee prosthesis which became painful. No intracellular material is visible. Haematoxylin–eosin × 400. (b) Same field as (a), viewed between crossed polars. Shows diffuse mottled birefringence of small intracellular particles of polyethylene. (The dust particles are in fact in the mounting medium.)

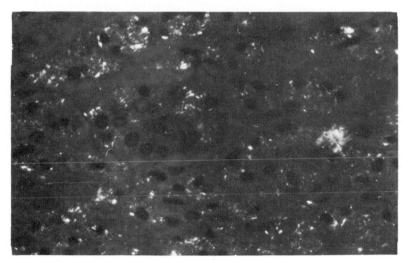

When ordinary light microscopy is combined with polarised light microscopy, it may be seen that the macrophages and giant cells contain variable quantities of intracellular foreign material. The foreign material which may be visualised is of three types (Vernon-Roberts and Freeman 1976) (Table 4.1): (1) *Metal-containing particles* are discrete and distinct black or brown-black granules, rods and needles up to 3 μm in maximum length (Fig. 4.15a) which are strongly birefringent when viewed between crossed polars (Fig. 4.15b); (2) *Polyethylene particles* are not visible in ordinary transmitted light but are strongly birefringent when viewed between crossed polars. The presence of smaller particles may be revealed by a diffuse mottled intracytoplasmic birefringence (Fig. 4.16), but larger fragments are in the form of granules, spears, splinters, ovoids and rectangles up to 50 μm in maximum dimension (Fig. 4.17); (3) *Acrylic cement fragments* are commonly seen, sometimes in large quantity, the size of the fragments varying up to several millimetres in maximum dimension. They are also frequently seen in the form of 'acrylic pearls' which may be clustered together and are frequently embedded in fibrous tissue (Fig. 4.18) with each pearl having a diameter of up to 80 μm. The cement fragments and acrylic pearls produce a predominantly giant cell reaction with each piece of cement surrounded by giant cells forming a syncytium having ill-defined cell boundaries. Cement particles may also be present as granules, splinters and irregular fragments surrounded by giant cells. Polymethylmethacrylate is distinguished from metal-containing particles and from polyethylene particles by the fact that it is readily soluble in the solvents used in normal tissue-processing procedures and its location in the tissues is therefore usually inferred from empty spaces in the tissues and cells. When present, cement is only very weakly birefringent when viewed between crossed polars.

The macrophages and giant cells also frequently contain large amounts of iron which becomes visible when sections are stained using the Perls technique. Winter (1974) carried out a visual assessment of the iron content in the tissues from around 44 cobalt–chromium and 44 stainless steel implants, and came to the conclusion that about 50 per cent of the cobalt–chromium cases contained iron to a minor degree only, while 75 per cent of the stainless steel cases contained iron which was frequently present in large amounts. He concluded that haemosiderin-like granules were a specific feature of the tissue reaction to stainless steel implants in a high proportion of cases, since he did not find haemosiderin-like granules in the tissues reacting to cobalt–chromium. By contrast, Vernon-Roberts and Freeman (1976) frequently found very large amounts of iron in the macrophages of the tissue reaction to both cobalt–chromium and stainless steel implants, and found haemosiderin-like granules in the tissues around cobalt–chromium implants. These workers also found large amounts of iron in the macrophages reacting to polyethylene particles shed from metal-against-polyethylene prostheses despite the fact that analytical studies of the same tissues revealed that only very low levels of cobalt, chromium and nickel had been released from the metallic components. The significance of the frequent presence of large amounts of iron in the cellular reaction around prosthetic implants is not clear, but iron deposition could be the result of haemoglobin breakdown following bleeding due to operative trauma or, more likely, to repeated minor episodes of trauma to the articular tissues after implantation. A similar constant oozing of blood into the joint cavity is thought to be the reason why large amounts of iron, sometimes amounting to haemosiderosis of the tissues, are so frequently found in rheumatoid synovial tissues (Mowat and Hothersall 1968; Muirden and Senator 1968).

As far as it is possible to assess it using microscopic and analytical methods, the degree of macrophage and giant cell reaction in the joint tissues around prostheses depends upon the amount of foreign material present in the tissues. The factors determining the degree and extent of macrophage and giant cell proliferation may be related to the total mass, total surface area, mean surface area or mean particle size of the foreign particles. While the exact nature of the relationship remains to be determined, in tissue sections examined microscopically there is a clear direct correlation between the number of metallic and polyethylene particles and the number of macro-

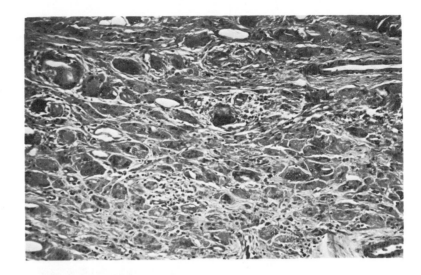

Figure 4.17.
(a) Many multinucleate giant cells and bands of fibrous tissue in articular tissues two years after implantation of a cobalt–chromium against high density polyethylene knee prosthesis which became painful and unstable. Haematoxylin–eosin × 120. (b) Same field as (a), viewed between crossed polars. Shows numerous birefringent fragments of polyethylene within giant cells and embedded in fibrous tissue. (The dust particles are in fact in the mounting medium.)

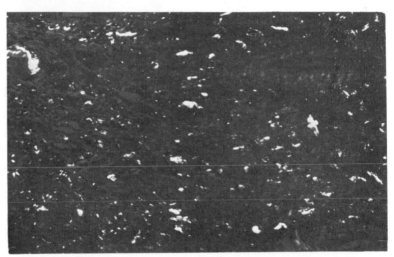

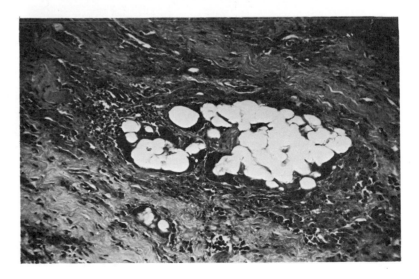

Figure 4.18.
Spaces representing site of cluster of 'acrylic pearls' of polymethylmethacrylate which is surrounded by syncytial giant cells and embedded in fibrous tissue in articular tissue around knee prosthesis. Haematoxylin–eosin × 120.

phages and giant cells present. Since foreign material having the morphological characteristics of metal-containing particles and polyethylene particles may be found within lymph nodes draining the region of a prosthesis (Fig. 4.19), it seems probable that at least some of the foreign particulate material is mobilised away from the articular tissues in normal circumstances. Thus it may be envisaged that in most patients who have asymptomatic functioning prostheses, a state of equilibrium is achieved in which the amount of foreign material being formed by the prosthesis and inducing a macrophage and giant cell reaction in the articular tissues is balanced by the replacement of cells by fibrous tissue and by the mobilisation of foreign material to lymph nodes. When large amounts of foreign material are generated, the macrophage and giant cell reaction is intensified so that all, or almost all, of the articular tissues are involved in the reaction and the state of equilibrium is lost. Histologically, the appearances suggest that equilibrium is lost more

Figure 4.19.
(a) Macrophages of corticomedullary sinus of iliac lymph node from patient who died 18 months after implantation of a cobalt–chromium against high density polyethylene knee prosthesis which was stable and painless. The macrophages contain black metallic-type particles. Haematoxylin–eosin × 400.
(b) Same field as (a), viewed between crossed polars. Shows that both metallic and polyethylene particles are present in the cells. (The dust particles are in fact in the mounting medium.)

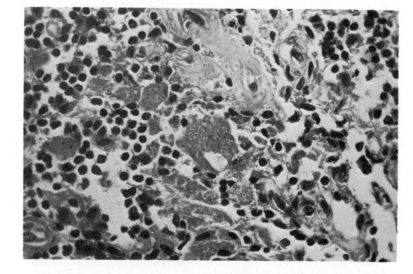

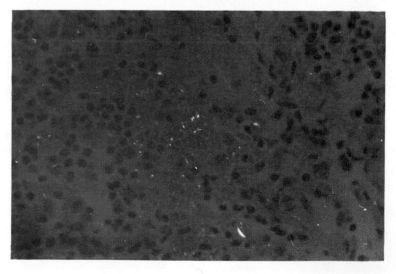

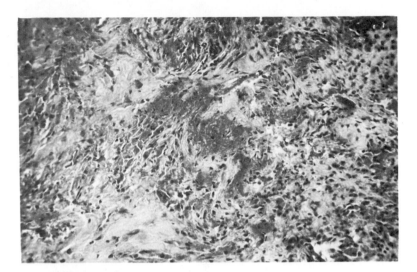

Figure 4.20.
Scattered areas of necrosis in articular granulation tissue four years after implantation of an all-cobalt–chromium hinged knee prosthesis which became loose. Haematoxylin–eosin × 120.

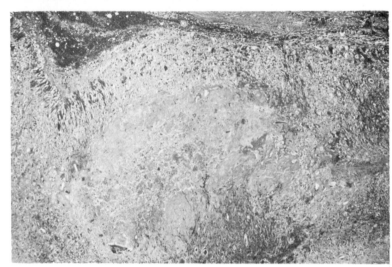

Figure 4.21.
Extensive necrosis of articular granulation tissue nine years after implantation of an all-cobalt–chromium hip prosthesis which had been increasingly painful for two years. Haematoxylin–eosin × 50.

rapidly in the face of the release of metal particles than in the face of the release of polyethylene; i.e. the latter appears to be more innocuous than the former (see section 4.1.1). In cases where there is abundant foreign material and an extensive cellular reaction, areas of necrosis in the reacting tissue are a frequent microscopic finding. These areas of necrosis may be small and scattered or extensive and diffuse (Figs. 4.20 and 4.21) and may involve areas of collagenised fibrous tissue in addition to macrophages and giant cells. The extensive breakdown of these tissues may result in the formation of pultaceous white or grey necrotic tissue, similar to caseous tuberculous debris, filling the joint cavity.

The position regarding the use of the recently introduced prostheses having bearing surfaces made from ceramic materials cannot yet be evaluated since there is no information available concerning the long-term effects of ceramic particles on human tissue during long-term use. Experience with other prosthetic materials has shown that caution must be exercised in predicting the outcome in clinical use of materials which function well in laboratory simulators and appear non-toxic in experimental studies. Nevertheless such experimental data as there are suggest that ceramic particles are biologically inert (Griss et al. 1973).

The topics of loosening and pain and their relationship to the histological response to wear debris are discussed in section 4.1 of this chapter.

3.2 Ultrastructural and Analytical Studies of Intracellular Crystalline Material in the Tissues Adjacent to Joint Prostheses

There is a dearth of published information regarding the electron microscopical appearances of the tissues around prostheses. Winter (1974) described very small fragments of highly crystalline foreign material in phagosomes within macrophages in the tissue surrounding an all-cobalt–chromium total hip prosthesis, and the Debye–Scherrer diffraction patterns were interpreted as indicating that the material was composed of unchanged cobalt–chromium alloy particles. In two other tissue samples from around all-cobalt–chromium knee and elbow prostheses, Winter (1974) found very small intracytoplasmic agglomerates having diffraction patterns which indicated that they were composed of carbides of chromium and cobalt. Vernon-Roberts and Freeman (1976) have observed similar very small electron-dense particles in the tissues around all-cobalt–chromium prostheses (later confirmed to contain cobalt and chromium by electron microscope microanalysis) but their size was such that they could not be responsible for the (relatively much larger) metal-containing crystalline particles visible by ordinary light microscopy and described earlier in this chapter. However, they observed intracytoplasmic electron-lucent crystalline structures (Fig. 4.22) having approximately the same dimensions as the metal-containing particles seen by light microscopy. Vernon-Roberts and Freeman (1976) also carried out electron microscopy of tissues containing abundant particles of high density polyethylene and found irregular plates of crystalline material (Fig. 4.23) which conformed with the shapes and sizes of polyethylene particles examined by polarised light microscopy.

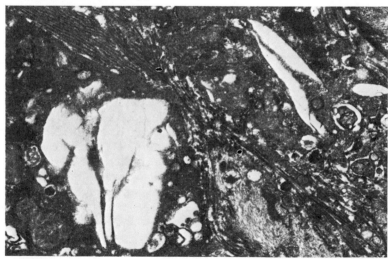

Figure 4.22.
Electron-lucent foreign material within macrophages in articular granulation tissue around an all-cobalt–chromium knee prosthesis which had become loose with extensive bone loss nine years after implantation. Light microscopy had revealed the presence of numerous black intracelluar crystalline particles of 'metallic' type in the granulation tissue. Electron micrograph × 15,000.

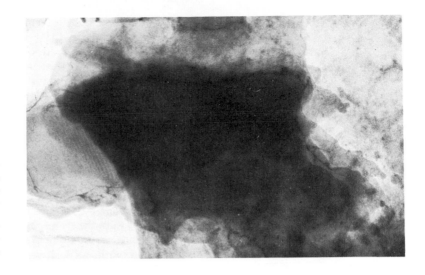

Figure 4.23.
Moderately electron-dense crystalline material within macrophage in articular granulation tissue around a cobalt–chrome against high density polyethylene knee prosthesis implanted for 15 months and which had become painful. Polarised light microscopy had revealed the presence of abundant intracellular particles of 'polyethylene' type. Electron micrograph × 50,000.

Vernon-Roberts and Freeman (1976) carried out preliminary electron microscope microanalysis (EMMA) of the intracytoplasmic foreign particles visible in the light microscope. In four patients who had very high concentrations of cobalt, chromium or nickel in the articular tissues analysed by neutron activation analysis (NAA), and in which the same articular tissues had numerous black intracellular particles when examined by light microscopy, EMMA of the particles demonstrated the presence of nickel, iron and titanium in all four cases; by contrast, in two patients having much lower concentrations of metal in the articular tissues analysed by NAA, and in which the same tissues contained large amounts of polyethylene particles when examined by polarised light microscopy, EMMA showed that nickel and iron were absent from the particles. The finding of titanium in most tissues examined by EMMA, despite its absence from the alloys used in the manufacture of most total joint replacement prostheses, is not surprising in view of the EMMA finding of trace amounts in the tissues of persons who have never had any form of metal implant (Henderson, personal communication 1975). It is of interest that Vernon-Roberts and Freeman (1976) were unable to detect the presence of cobalt in any of the crystals examined by EMMA in any of their six cases, and Semlitsch, Vogel and Willert (1972) also found virtually no cobalt or chromium in the connective tissues around all-metal hip prostheses using electron probe microanalysis (EPMA), but this was not the case for hip joints in which a metallic ball articulated with a mica-reinforced PTFE socket.

The variable presence of chromium, and the complete absence of detectable cobalt in EMMA studies of the intracellular particles visible in the light microscope (Vernon-Roberts and Freeman 1976), despite the NAA findings of high levels of one or both elements in the same tissues as a whole in some cases, could be accounted for by the high solubility of cobalt and chromium compounds resulting in their removal from the intracellular crystals during the processing of tissues for electron microscopy (although analytical studies have tended to exclude this possibility) or by the postulate that they normally exist as sub-light microscopic particles (such as have been observed by Winter (1974) and by Vernon-Roberts and Freeman (1976)) or as soluble salts of cobalt and chromium. Until further EMMA and EPMA studies are carried out, all that can be said is that, although numerous metal-containing particles are visible, using light microscopy, in the tissues around all-cobalt–chromium prostheses, cobalt and chromium do not appear to contribute to the formation of these crystalline particles (at least not in every case). By contrast, the EMMA results available indicate a more important role for nickel in the formation of these structures. Nickel is present in a concentration of 10–15 per cent in stainless steel and its presence in the tissues around stainless steel prostheses is not surprising: however, no more than 2·5 per cent nickel is permitted in the specification of cast cobalt–chromium alloy, and the amount actually present is often less than this. The presence of nickel in significant quantities in the tissues and its invariable presence in the particles around cobalt–chromium as well as stainless steel prostheses supports the view that the metal detectable in the articular tissues and in intra-cytoplasmic particles is not simply wear debris but rather the end result of wear, corrosion, chemical interaction with other substances (for example, protein) and phagocytosis (Vernon-Roberts, Freeman and Sculco, in preparation).

4 THE ROLE OF THE TISSUE RESPONSE TO IMPLANTS AND THEIR WEAR PRODUCTS IN THE CAUSATION OF THE COMPLICATIONS OF TOTAL JOINT REPLACEMENTS

Certain complications may mar the functional result following joint replacement. These include loosening, infection, pain in the absence of both loosening and infection, and (theoretically at least) neoplasia. Obviously all of these complications may be caused by factors which have nothing to do with the tissue response to the implant itself or to its wear products. In some cases, however, it seems possible that variations in the normal tissue response may be partly or wholly responsible. In the following sections the possible connections between the tissue response and these complications will be explored.

4.1 Loosening

4.1.1 LOOSENING IN THE ABSENCE OF TISSUE SENSITIVITY TO IMPLANT MATERIALS

It seems possible that two events of a biological nature may be involved in the genesis of prosthetic loosening: bone death and the tissue response to debris.

Bone Death

In our experience (Vernon-Roberts and Freeman 1976) early loosening (i.e. loosening within two years of implantation) is usually associated with the death of more bone than appears to be the case with non-loose prostheses which have been implanted for the same period of time. This association between bone death and loosening suggests a causal relationship.

Firstly, it seems possible that the sequence of events discussed in section 2.2 of this chapter as leading to fracture of dead bone at the interface may lead to an actual loss of the interlock between living bone and cement rather than merely to fibrous replacement of a zone of dead bone.

Secondly, the death of a substantial zone of bone adjacent to the implant might result, over a period of years, in the development of an unusually thick layer of fibrous tissue (Fig. 4.12) at the bone–cement interface (for reasons discussed in section 2.2 of this chapter), which it seems reasonable to think would be exposed to tensile and shear stresses in a way from which a narrower zone would be protected since the narrower is the zone of fibrous tissue, the more irregularities on the bones themselves interlock. Since soft connective tissue is relatively weak in tension and shear (and indeed responds to repeated shear stresses by cavity formation, as in adventitious bursae), this again may predispose to loosening (by rupture of the fibrous tissue rather than by fracture of the bone). Support for this view comes from the fact that Willert, Ludwig and Semlitsch (1974) have observed tears, haemorrhages and fibrinous exudates in the fibrous tissue of the permanent implant bed in cases of loosening occurring more than two years after implantation.

Thus excessive bone death may predispose to early or late loosening, especially in heavily loaded bone–prosthesis interfaces, either because the dead bone fractures, leading to relatively early loosening, or because a thick zone of fibrous tissue ruptures, leading to loosening of the prosthesis at a later stage.

It must be emphasised that cleft formation in the fibrous bed of an implant may not always lead to excessive, clinically evident movement because cleft formation does not necessarily mean that the bony interlock is lost. Indeed, arthrographic examination of symptomless prostheses frequently shows the presence of such clefts (Murray and Rodrigo 1975) and Vernon-Roberts and Freeman (in preparation) have found focally high concentrations of polyethylene particles in the fibrous tissue implant bed of many prostheses, indicating the existence of clefts (such as those which Murray demonstrated arthrographically) extending from the synovial cavity. It seems possible that the accumulation of polyethylene wear debris in such clefts may lead to necrosis of the fibrous tissue in the implant bed, in the same way as such particles may lead to tissue necrosis elsewhere (see section 3.1 of this chapter). This in turn may convert a symptomless prosthesis, with cleft formation in its fibrous bed but without material movement between bone and implant, into a symptomatic prosthesis with substantial movement. This sequence of events may also be relevant to the development of pain in the absence of loosening (see section 4.3).

Once a cemented implant has become loose, movement of the cement against the bone abrades the cement and the bone undergoes resorption. The result is the production of an expanded cavity within the bone filled with pultaceous material composed of fragmented cement and dead tissue. It is relatively easy to see how pain may be produced in this situation: bone has a rich nerve supply, and the fragmentation of both living and dead bone could well give rise to pain of bony origin. Localised high stresses on the bone produced by a loss of contact over much of the bone–implant interface may also play a part in the production of pain.

The Tissue Response to Debris

A second pathological process leading to loosening is suggested if the current information regarding the histopathology and tissue metal concentrations (see Table 4.3) in patients whose prostheses loosen more than two years after implantation is considered as a whole. This, as yet hypothetical, chain of events is illustrated diagrammatically in Figs. 4.24, 4.25 and 4.30, and is outlined below.

All prostheses having bearing surfaces release wear products into the joint cavity surrounding the articulating components (Fig. 4.24). Metal-on-metal prostheses frequently release abundant metal, metal-on-bone prostheses release lesser amounts of metal, and metal-on-plastic prostheses usually release very small amounts of metal. High density polyethylene bearing surfaces normally release only very small amounts of plastic, but occasionally abundant wear particles of plastic are formed. Metal is released from prostheses by corrosion, and there is almost certainly rapid corrosion of metallic wear particles. Thus, under normal circumstances, there are variable amounts of metal and/or plastic wear particles and metal salts within the joint cavity surrounding a prosthesis.

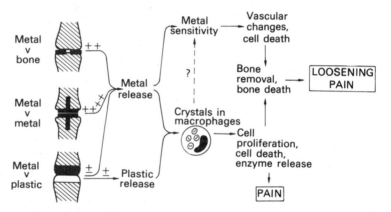

Figure 4.24.
Diagram to illustrate possible sequence of events leading to pain and loosening.

Crystalline structures containing metal or composed of plastic wear particles appear within macrophages and giant cells of the articular tissues (Fig. 4.24). The larger the amount of either of these crystalline materials that is formed, the greater is the extent of macrophage and giant cell proliferation. While the plastic wear particles are ingested by the phagocytic cells and remain in unchanged form, metal-containing crystals appear to be formed within the phagocytic cells from the metal salts arising from corrosion of bearing surfaces and metallic wear particles (i.e. they are not themselves the wear particles in unchanged form).

When crystalline particles of metal or plastic are present in large amounts, there is frequently evidence of cell and tissue death. Tissue death is particularly marked when abundant metal is present in the tissues, and this may be related to the presence of cobalt salts which do not appear to participate in crystal formation but probably exist as soluble salts in solution. It is already known that there are certain exceptions to the generally harmless effects of the phagocytosis of inorganic materials by macrophages; thus it is well established that silica particles are intensely toxic to macrophages and kill them during a process in which the phagolysosomes containing the silica

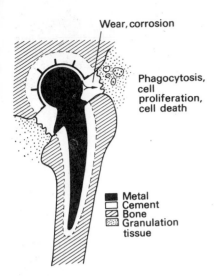

Wear, corrosion

Phagocytosis,
cell
proliferation,
cell death

■ Metal
□ Cement
▨ Bone
▨ Granulation
tissue

Figure 4.25.
Diagram illustrating proliferation of macrophages and giant cells in articular tissues in response to products of wear and corrosion.

particles rupture and release the lysosomal enzymes into the cell cytoplasm (Allison, Harington and Birbeck 1966). After death the macrophages containing silica disintegrate and the material is re-phagocytosed; the cycle is then repeated and a strong stimulus to fibrogenesis is exerted. If intracellular particles containing metal (and, to a lesser degree, plastic wear particles) have a similar effect, particularly when present in large numbers, this could account for the death of cells and tissues around some prostheses (Fig. 4.25). Evidence supporting a toxic effect of particulate metals on macrophages has recently been provided by Rae (1975), who found that particulate cobalt, nickel and cobalt–chromium alloy (produced in the laboratory from total joint replacement prostheses articulating in a joint simulator) were toxic to mouse macrophages *in vitro*, while titanium, chromium and molybdenum particles were well tolerated by these cells. In the majority of cases in which loosening is present, macrophages and giant cells containing abundant foreign material have extended into the bone forming the implant bed (Figs. 4.26 and 4.27). Although the possibility must be considered that this cellular

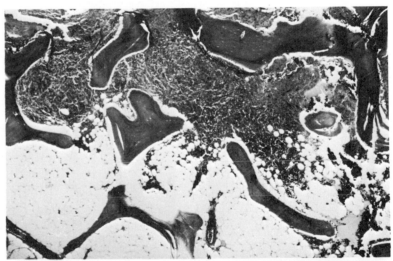

Figure 4.26.
Granulation tissue extending from articular tissue into periarticular bone four years after implantation of an all-cobalt–chromium hinged knee prosthesis which became loose. Haematoxylin–eosin × 50.

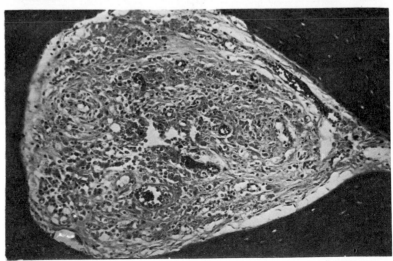

Figure 4.27.
Granulation tissue with numerous macrophages containing metallic particles occupying a vascular channel in the cortical bone of the femur adjacent to a loose cobalt–chromium-against-bone hip prosthesis 14 years after implantation. The bone is dead. Haematoxylin–eosin × 120.

Figure 4.28.
Living and dead periarticular bone being removed by infiltrating granulation tissue four years after implantation of an all-cobalt–chromium hinged knee prosthesis which became loose. Haematoxylin–eosin × 120.

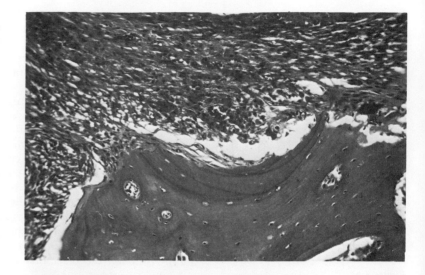

Figure 4.29.
Death and disappearance of cortical and cancellous bone and its replacement by partly necrotic granulation tissue in femur 14 years after implantation of cobalt–chromium-against-bone hip prosthesis which became loose. Haematoxylin–eosin × 50.

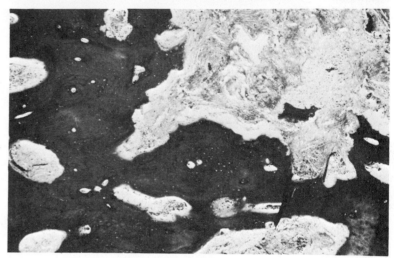

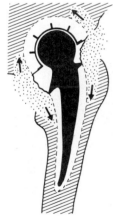

Bone removal, bone death, bone replaced by granulation tissue, death of granulation tissue

↓

LOOSENING
OF
PROSTHESIS

Figure 4.30.
Diagram illustrating how loosening of prosthesis arises from the extension of articular granulation tissue into the bone and from the removal of bone around the cement which bonds the prosthesis in position.

extension follows loosening, the appearances suggest that the proliferating cells may first enter the marrow spaces of the cancellous bone nearest to the articulation without initial loss of the bone (Fig. 4.26), and that active removal of both living and dead trabecular bone by the infiltrating tissues occurs later (Fig. 4.28); i.e. that infiltration precedes loosening rather than that loosening precedes infiltration. The infiltrating tissues eventually enter the Haversian canals of compact bone, cause bone death by interference with the blood supply, and remove both dead and living compact bone by active resorption (Fig. 4.29). The removal of bone from the implant bed and its replacement by non-osseous soft tissue must result in the loss of the osseous anchors necessary for the firm fixation of the cement bonding the prosthesis into the bone and it would seem that this must in turn predispose to loosening (Fig. 4.30). Since the macrophages and giant cells invading the bone are an extension of the reaction taking place in the joint tissues, it follows that the bone which is first invaded and then removed is the bone nearest to the articulation. Thus prostheses fixed by intramedullary stems become unsupported near the articulation while the remainder of the stem may still be firmly anchored in place: a situation which may result in fracture of the stem because of the excessive stresses placed upon it (Chapter 2).

In summary, it appears that:

(1) a direct correlation exists between the amount of particulate foreign material present and the degree of macrophage and giant cell reaction in the articular tissues surrounding an implant;

(2) the greater the degree of macrophage and giant cell proliferation in the articular tissues, the greater is the tendency towards the invasion and replacement of bone by the proliferating cells; and

(3) invasion and removal of bone resulting from this cellular infiltration seems likely to lead to progressive loosening of the prosthesis.

Thus the histological evidence suggests that the amount of particulate foreign material present in the articular tissues may be a factor in determining whether a prosthesis remains firmly fixed or becomes loose.

4.1.2 LOOSENING IN THE PRESENCE OF TISSUE SENSITIVITY TO IMPLANT MATERIALS

It is widely recognised that the skin may become sensitive to various metals applied to the skin surface and that this sensitivity can be detected by epicutaneous patch tests in which a positive response is denoted by an eczematous reaction occurring when a solution of the relevant metal is placed on the skin. Since falsely negative results may occur with epicutaneous patch tests of this sort, more reliable results may be obtained by studying the reaction to intracutaneously injected solutions of metal salts, particularly in the case of trivalent chromium (Fregert and Rorsman 1966a). Cobalt, chromium and nickel are all capable of exciting skin sensitivity. The readiness with which sensitivity can be induced and demonstrated with each of these three elements depends upon the solubility of the element in the form presented to the tissue, and thus upon the nature of the anion when the element is presented as a salt or upon the nature of the alloy when it is presented as the metal (Fregert and Rorsman 1966a, b). Although the incidence of skin sensitivity to cobalt, chromium and nickel in the general population is unknown, in a group of 5 416 subjects suspected of having contact dermatitis, Fregert and Rorsman (1966b) found an incidence of epicutaneous sensitivity in women to nickel of 2·5 per cent, to cobalt of 1·7 per cent and to chromium of 0·8 per cent; and, by contrast, men displayed an incidence of sensitivity to chromium of 3·8 per cent, to cobalt of 1·6 per cent and to nickel of 0·9 per cent.

The presence of skin sensitivity after the insertion of non-articulating metal implants in the tissues has been described in four cases of dermatitis developing in patients who had pins or plates inserted (Laugier and Foussereau 1966), a case of dermatitis due to sensitivity to a cobalt–chromium denture (Brendlinger and Tarsitano 1970), and a case of urticaria following the insertion of a cobalt–chromium nail for a femoral fracture (McKenzie, Aitken and Risdill-Smith 1967).

An association between late loosening of prostheses for the total replacement of a joint and demonstrable epicutaneous skin sensitivity to metal was first described by Evans et al. (1974). Their results, and those of other workers, are summarised in Table 4.2. They found (Table 4.2) that of a total of 14 patients having loose prostheses, 9 had positive skin sensitivity tests to metal (7 to cobalt, 1 to chromium, and 1 to both nickel and cobalt); by contrast, 24 patients with normally functioning, securely fixed prostheses were not sensitive to metal. The findings suggested that there was a strong association between metal sensitivity and loosening of prostheses composed entirely of cobalt–chromium alloy. These findings received support from the studies of Jones et al. (1975) who found positive skin sensitivity to cobalt in 6 patients having late failure of all-cobalt–chromium McKee hip prostheses, and negative skin tests in 30 patients in whom McKee hip prostheses were functioning satisfactorily. Benson, Goodwin and Brostoff (1975) have also confirmed that there is an unexpectedly high incidence of skin sensitivity to cobalt and chromium in patients with metal-to-metal prostheses. They found that 9 (28 per cent) of a total of 32 patients with McKee hip prostheses were sensitive to metal (1 to nickel alone, 2 to both nickel and cobalt, 3 to cobalt alone, and 3 to chromium alone), while only 1 (2·6 per cent) of a total of 39 patients with metal-to-high density polyethylene Charnley hip prostheses was sensitive to nickel. Three (9·1 per cent) of a total of 33 control patients awaiting total hip replacement were sensitive (2 to nickel alone, and 1 to nickel and cobalt in combination). Two of the McKee prostheses failed because of loosening, and both patients gave positive reactions to chromium alone. In another study, Elves et al. (1975) investigated a total of 50 patients who were recipients of various types of total joint replacements, and found skin sensitivity to metal in 19 cases (38 per cent) (2 to nickel alone, 8 to cobalt alone, 6 to both cobalt and nickel, 1 to both nickel and vanadium, and 2 to chromium). In 23 of the patients non-traumatic failure of the prosthesis had occurred, and 15 of these patients were sensitive to metal; out of the remaining 27 patients with no evidence of loosening, 4 were sensitive to nickel and cobalt or to cobalt alone.

The clinical studies of epicutaneous skin sensitivity to metal in patients having joint prostheses therefore clearly show that after the implantation of a prosthesis in which cobalt–chromium articulates with cobalt–chromium certain patients are sensitive to cobalt, and less frequently to chromium or nickel. Sensitivity may also be present

Table 4.2   Incidence of Skin Sensitivity to Metal in Patients With Joint Endoprostheses—Results From Various Sources

Reference	Number of patients tested	Stable prostheses			Loose prostheses		
		Number	Number sensitive	Percentage sensitive	Number	Number sensitive	Percentage sensitive
Evans et al. (1974)	38	24	0	0	14	9	64
Jones et al. (1975)	37	30	0	0	7	6	86
Benson, Goodwin and Brostoff (1975)	72	70	10	14	2	2	100
Elves et al. (1975)	50	27	4	15	23	15	65
Aggregated results	197	151	14	9	46	32	70

in patients having prostheses in which cobalt–chromium articulates against bone (Evans et al. 1974), but the incidence of sensitivity in patients with metal-against-plastic prostheses does not, on the basis of present evidence, appear to be higher than in controls not having prostheses (Benson, Goodwin and Brostoff 1975). The findings do not allow a definite distinction to be made between the possibilities that: (1) the patients were metal-sensitive before implantation of the prosthesis; (2) the patients became sensitive after implantation of the prosthesis; or (3) that one or other sequence was common to all cases. However, the strikingly higher incidence of metal sensitivity in patients with metal-on-metal prostheses compared with the much lower incidence in patients with metal-on-plastic prostheses and in control subjects indicates that metal sensitivity is the result of the much higher concentrations of metallic wear products generated by metal-on-metal prostheses compared with the considerably smaller amounts generated by metal-on-plastic prostheses (Coleman, Herrington and Scales 1973; Swanson, Freeman and Heath 1973; Evans et al. 1974; Vernon-Roberts and Freeman 1976). Moreover, the most significant finding in these studies of skin sensitivity in patients with joint prostheses would appear to be the very high incidence of skin sensitivity to cobalt alone, since sensitivity to cobalt alone is rare in dermatological practice (i.e. in patients without prostheses) when compared to the comparatively common positive reactions to nickel alone or nickel and cobalt in combination (Fregert and Rorsman 1966b). Since it is highly unlikely that sensitivity to cobalt alone (or a predisposition to the development of sensitivity to cobalt alone) induces susceptibility to the more severe forms of joint disease leading to joint replacement, the frequency of sensitivity to cobalt alone in patients with prostheses clearly indicates that cobalt sensitivity develops *after* the prosthesis is inserted in the majority of cases.

The other highly significant finding in these studies is the very high incidence of metal sensitivity in patients with unexplained loosening of prostheses, and this suggests that there is a causal relationship between metal sensitivity and loosening. A number of controlled prospective studies using epicutaneous skin testing are in progress, both in patients having prostheses functioning satisfactorily and in patients before arthroplasty has been performed. Since it is conceivable that the patch testing procedure itself could lead to sensitisation, it would seem to be unwise to perform this investigation frequently in the same patient as a routine preimplantation or postimplantation procedure. Lymphocytes from patients with nickel or chromium sensitivity have been shown to undergo blastic transformation *in vitro* in the presence of salts of the appropriate metal under certain conditions, and it is to be hoped that current attempts to perfect similar *in vitro* tests using lymphocytes from patients with joint prostheses will result in a safe method of detecting pre- and postimplant metal sensitivity, particularly to cobalt.

Histopathological studies of articular tissues from patients having loosening and metal sensitivity (Evans et al. 1974; Jones et al. 1975; Vernon-Roberts and Freeman 1976) have revealed extensive necrosis of tissues and a very marked proliferation of macrophages and giant cells containing large amounts of intracellular metal-containing particles. This group of patients also tend to have very marked

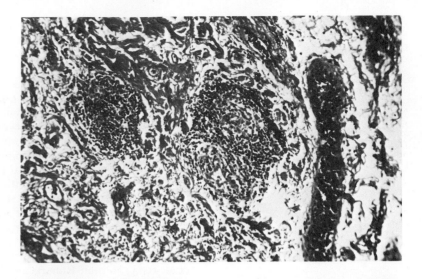

Figure 4.31.
(a) Lymphocytic vasculitis and degenerate connective tissue in articular tissue of patient sensitive to cobalt. Haematoxylin–eosin × 120. (b) Fibrinoid necrosis of arterioles in articular connective tissues of patient sensitive to cobalt. Haematoxylin–eosin × 120. (c) Articular connective tissue showing obliteration of lumen of large and small arteries by fibrous intimal proliferation in patient sensitive to cobalt. Haematoxylin–eosin × 120.

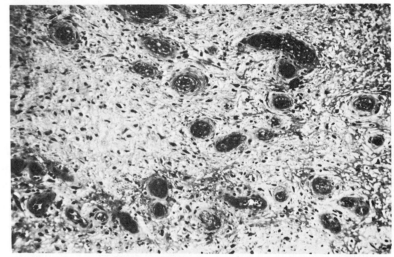

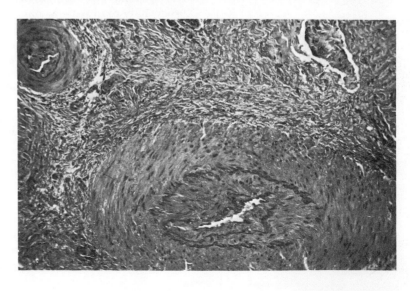

obliterative vascular changes in the form of lymphocytic vasculitis, fibrinoid necrosis and fibrous intimal proliferation (Fig. 4.31). While some of these changes could be secondary to tissue degeneration and death, their presence in tissues still alive or undergoing early degenerative changes indicates that the death of these tissues may be partly or largely due to the deprivation of their blood supply. In this group of patients, the invasion of bone by macrophages and giant cells is generally widespread with extensive death of the invading tissues and of the bone, fragmentation of the cement, and abundant necrotic debris within the joint cavity.

There is evidence, therefore, that in patients with metal sensitivity the tissue reaction to the products of wear and corrosion is exaggerated, tissue death is associated with large amounts of foreign intracellular material and obliterative changes in blood vessels, bone death and replacement by proliferating macrophages and giant cells are rapid and widespread, and that the condition is progressive while the prosthesis remains implanted.

Since there is evidence of a relationship between metal sensitivity and metal-on-metal implants, it is necessary to examine the tissue metal concentrations in relation to different types of prosthesis to ascertain whether the rate of release of metal differs in sensitive and non-sensitive patients. Studies of metal concentration in the tissues adjacent to loose prostheses by Evans et al. (1974) showed that the tissues around five cobalt–chromium-on-cobalt–chromium prostheses (four patients) contained very high concentrations of both cobalt and chromium; cobalt and chromium concentrations were also elevated in the tissues around three cobalt–chromium-on-bone prostheses, although not to the levels seen with cobalt–chromium-on-cobalt–chromium prostheses; much lower concentrations of cobalt and chromium, approaching the levels seen in controls, were found in the tissues around three prostheses in which cobalt–chromium articulated against high density polyethylene. Later results (Vernon-Roberts, Freeman and Sculco, in preparation) confirm and extend the above findings. They show (Table 4.3) that cobalt, chromium and nickel levels are markedly elevated in the tissues around cobalt–chromium-on-bone prostheses but to much lower levels than is the case with cobalt–chromium-on-cobalt–chromium prostheses, while generally low levels of all three metals are found in the tissues

Table 4.3 Concentration of Cobalt, Chromium and Nickel Measured by Neutron Activation Analysis of Tissues Adjacent to Painful or Loose Prostheses

Articulating surfaces of prosthesis	Number of patients	Parts per million in tissue: average and range		
		Cobalt	Chromium	Nickel
Cobalt–chromium on cobalt–chromium	8	43·1 (11–230)	57·2 (18–103)	2·3 (0·1–6·0)
Cobalt–chromium on bone	9	0·7 (0·02–2·5)	3·4 (0·12–9·3)	4·0 (0·3–20)
Cobalt–chromium on polyethylene	9	0·56 (0·02–2·2)	0·86 (0·15–2·0)	0·31 (0·2–0·6)
Stainless steel on polyethylene	12	0·06 (0·01–0·5)	0·56 (0·06–1·3)	0·76 (0·1–2·0)

around prostheses in which cobalt–chromium or stainless steel articulates against high density polyethylene. The findings indicate that the higher metal levels are present in those patients who also exhibit skin sensitivity. While it is not clear whether skin sensitivity precedes or follows the accumulation of high concentrations of metal, the available evidence suggests that the presence of metal in high concentration leads to sensitisation rather than vice versa. The fact that loosening is not restricted to patients having high concentrations of metal in the articular tissues indicates that a direct toxic effect of high concentrations of metals on the tissues is unlikely to be the only factor (if it is a factor at all) inducing tissue death.

The following practical implications appertaining to patient management follow from these conclusions.

(1) Since the rate of release of cobalt, chromium and nickel is much higher from prostheses in which cobalt–chromium articulates against cobalt–chromium, it appears advisable to use metal-against-polyethylene prostheses whenever possible on the basis of metal concentrations in the tissues. On this basis, stainless steel and cobalt–chromium are equally acceptable articulating against polyethylene.

(2) All patients in whom prostheses become loose should be tested for metal sensitivity. If they are found to be sensitive, loosening may be expected to be progressive and removal of the prosthesis is indicated.

(3) It is desirable that a safe non-sensitising method (probably therefore an *in vitro* method) should be available for assessing sensitivity to cobalt, chromium and nickel. Ideally this should be carried out before implantation of an alloy containing one of these metals so as to avoid implanting a metal to which the patient is sensitive (both cobalt–chromium and stainless steel contain chromium and nickel). In practice, this point may not be of great value if a metal-on-polyethylene prosthesis is to be used.

(4) Tissue necrosis is marked in many patients with loose prostheses associated with metal sensitivity, and this leads to the formation of abundant necrotic pultaceous debris within the joint cavity and around the loose prosthesis. Hitherto, this necrotic tissue has often been regarded as evidence for the presence of infection although no pathogenic organism is cultured. The figures currently quoted in the literature for the incidence of infection may therefore require re-examination and revision. Moreover, some cases of true infection may represent secondary infection of necrotic debris resulting from metal sensitivity.

4.2 Infection

Clearly, infection around an implant depends in the first place upon whether bacteria reach the operative wound. However, even if the wound does become contaminated, wound sepsis will not inevitably follow since invading bacteria will be destroyed by host defence mechanisms provided the tissues are healthy. Thus as Freeman (1975) has pointed out, there are a number of ways in which prosthetic design may influence the outcome of bacterial contamination. First, host defence mechanisms may have limited access to the interface region between the implant and its bed, and a prosthesis should therefore have as small an external surface as possible compatible with the need for secure bonding to bone. Second, since host defence mechanisms can only operate in living vascularised tissues, care should be taken to limit bone death to the minimum at the time of implantation and haematomata should be avoided by ensuring that 'dead spaces' around the implant are not present. Third, steps should be taken to reduce operative exposure of the tissues to a minimum. If, in spite of these precautions, infection develops and the prosthesis has to be removed, prosthetic design should be such as to make removal easy and conversion to an acceptable alternative (for example, arthrodesis) possible. While these considerations relating to operative technique and prosthetic design are clearly of great importance in relation to infections which are apparent within the period up to a few months after operation, they may have a less important and indirect part to play in 'infections' occurring several months or years after implantation of the prosthesis.

In many instances, late pain or loosening have been ascribed to the presence of infection because exploration of the prosthesis has revealed the presence of 'purulent', 'caseous' or pultaceous matter inside the joint and around the stem of the prosthesis. However, bacteria cannot always be identified in tissue samples examined microbiologically. Histological examination of the pultaceous matter reveals that it is usually composed of necrotic connective tissues containing fragments of dead bone and, depending upon the type of prosthesis, may also contain metal-containing crystals or polyethylene particles (Evans et al. 1974; Vernon-Roberts and Freeman 1976). The reasons why the tissues die in the presence of foreign particles have been examined earlier in this chapter, and the reasons why tissue death tends to be more extensive in the presence of sensitivity to metal have also been stated: all the evidence points to the fact that the presence of abundant foreign particles liberated from some prostheses in some patients leads to widespread tissue death and the accumulation of necrotic tissue of the type which will be encountered at exploration of the 'infected' prosthesis. There is now also abundant evidence that such tissue death is more extensive when metal sensitivity is present due to the release of metal from metal-on-metal prostheses. This necrotic tissue is not pus nor the product of caseous necrosis (a type of necrosis restricted to tuberculous lesions), but, as dead tissue, it may provide the ideal medium for secondary infection. Although secondary infection seems likely in theory, in practice it appears to be uncommon since examination of the tissues from over 100 cases of late pain and loosening has not revealed a single case of proven infection (Vernon-Roberts and Freeman, work in progress). This suggests that the finding of pultaceous material around a prosthesis warrants not only microbiological examination of the material, but also careful examination of the tissues for evidence of metallic crystals or polyethylene particles, and tests for the presence of metal sensitivity. Unless pathogenic organisms are cultured and pus cells seen, it would seem unjustifiable to ascribe these episodes of late tissue breakdown to infection.

4.3 Pain in the Absence of Loosening and Infection

While, in the authors' experience, pain in the region of a prosthesis is usually due to loosening, to the presence of infection, or occasionally to factors outside the prosthesis such as Paget's disease of bone, metastatic tumour or the deposition of calcium pyrophosphate dihydrate crystals in synovial tissues, definite evidence of these pathological processes being the cause of the pain is sometimes lacking. Infection is often suspected but hardly ever confirmed by micro-biological evidence, and, apart from loosening, the other causes quoted above are so rarely found in practice that they may for practical purposes be ignored.

Examination of tissues removed from around stable but painful prostheses (Vernon-Roberts and Freeman 1976; Vernon-Roberts, Freeman and Sculco, work in progress) has revealed that the majority of these patients have variable amounts of metal-containing crystals or polyethylene particles, medium to low metal concentrations and evidence of cell and tissue death on a limited or wide scale in the articular tissues. Cell death in these cases predominantly affects the macrophages which have taken up the foreign particles. Macrophages contain abundant degradative enzymes contained within lysosomes, and their death is known (in other circumstances) to be associated with the release of these enzymes into surrounding tissues causing the death not only of other macrophages but also of other tissues such as fibrous tissue, bone, etc. Such joints might be painful because of the release of lysosomal enzymes following macrophage death (since these enzymes are thought to be capable of inducing pain in other circumstances) and pain could arise from the inflammation which is the inevitable sequel to tissue death in general.

4.4 Neoplasia

Exogenous agents which may lead to tumour formation may be chemical, physical or biological in nature. It is easy to see, therefore, how implanted materials used in joint replacement could, in principle, be implicated in the causation of tumours. Moreover, both the chemical and physical characteristics of the materials used could theoretically be held responsible. In this respect, it has been well established that metallic powders, metallic salts, and metallic wear particles (produced from joint prostheses in laboratory simulators) are all capable of producing malignant neoplasms when injected into rodents (Oppenheimer et al. 1956; Heath and Daniel 1962; Heath, Freeman and Swanson 1971). It has also been shown that various plastic materials, including polyethylene and polymethyl-methacrylate, are capable of inducing tumour formation in rodents (Oppenheimer et al. 1955). The relevance of all these experimental findings in rodents to tumour formation around implants in man is difficult to judge. Although a wide range of materials have been shown to be carcinogenic, this property seems to depend upon the shape of the implant rather than upon its chemistry, and fortunately the carcinogenic properties of plastics are much reduced or lost when they are implanted in powder form (Nothdurft 1955; Oppenheimer et al. 1955, 1959, 1961). It is now widely thought that the difference in carcinogenicity between different shapes of the same plastic depends upon whether or not the implant is encapsulated since tumours arise from the walls of the capsules (see Oppenheimer et al. 1959, and, for a review of the literature, Bischoff and Bryson 1964). Reassuringly, polyethylene implanted in particulate form does not become encapsulated experimentally and neither do wear particles of high density polyethylene released into the tissues from prostheses in the dog (Walker et al. 1974) and in man (Charosky, Bullough and Wilson 1973; Vernon-Roberts and Freeman, work in progress). In line with their failure to become encapsulated, polyethylene particles have not been found to induce tumours save in one study, that of Carter and Roe (1969) who were able to induce tumours with shredded polyethylene in the rat. In general, the carcinogenicity of plastics has been demonstrated repeatedly only in rodents and rarely in man, although the apparent immunity of man may perhaps be due to the length of the latent interval for tumour induction (Bischoff and Bryson 1964). Carter and Roe's study was stimulated by Cleland's experience that tumours had occurred in two patients treated for pulmonary tuberculosis by extraperiosteal plombage with PTFE on one occasion and hollow polyethylene spheres on a second (Cleland, personal communication 1974). The form in which polyethylene was implanted by Carter and Roe gave rise to a considerable and sustained local response (although not to encapsulation) and it may have been this fact which was responsible for tumour formation. Carter and Roe themselves comment that their material, which consisted of numerous shreds 8–9 mm long, behaved more like a sponge than a collection of particles. The polyethylene particles seen in the tissues around prostheses in man are widely separated from each other and are only 1–2 μm in diameter (Vernon-Roberts and Freeman, work in progress) so that physically they do not resemble the material implanted by Carter and Roe.

Over-all, therefore, the experimental observations currently available very strongly suggest that the particles of polyethylene which are shed from polyethylene prostheses in clinical use are not carcinogenic in animals or in man.

Thus at present both metal-on-metal (cobalt–chromium) and metal-on-plastic joint prostheses are known to wear *in vivo* and therefore to produce particles; such evidence as is available shows that the particles produced from all-cobalt–chromium prostheses are carcinogenic when injected in massive doses into the rat, and suggests indirectly that polyethylene wear particles are not carcinogenic in experimental animals. The exact relevance of this to joint replacement in practice is not clear.

According to Williams (1973) there is a minimum latent period for tumour formation, which is related to the life span of the species involved, and would therefore be expected to be considerably longer in man than in the mouse: perhaps up to 20 years or longer. In patients with joint replacement prostheses, the rate of liberation of wear particles is many orders of magnitude lower than the rates represented by doses used in experimental animals, and the effect of this difference is not known. It is not even certain that tumours can be induced in man by this means, and it seems certain, on the basis of present clinical experience, that if they can the induction period will be so long as not to affect a large fraction of the patients concerned. Nevertheless, if implant-induced tumours do become manifest in man, this would necessarily lead to a radical re-evaluation of the whole of our thinking regarding the suitability of implant materials and the types of tissue reactions which they provoke.

REFERENCES

Allison, A. C., Harington, J. S. and Birbeck, M. (1966) An examination of the cytotoxic effects of silica on macrophages. *Journal of Experimental Medicine* **124**, 141.

Benson, M. K. D., Goodwin, P. G. and Brostoff, J. (1975) Metal sensitivity in patients with joint replacement arthroplasties. *British Medical Journal* **4**, 374.

Biehl, G., Harms, J. and Hanser, U. (1974) Experimentelle Untersuchungen über die Wärmeentwicklung im Knochen bei der Polymerisation von Knochenzement. Intraoperative Temperaturmessungen bei normaler Blutzirkulation und in Blutleere. *Archiv für Orthopädische und Unfall-Chirurgie* **78**, 62.

Biehl, G., Harms, J. and Mäusle, E. (1975) Tierexperimentelle und histopathologische Untersuchungen über die Anpassungsvorgänge des Knochens nach der Implantation von 'Tragrippen-Endoprosthesen'. *Archiv für Orthopädische und Unfall-Chirurgie* **81**, 105.

Bischoff, F. and Bryson, G. (1964) Carcinogenesis through solid state surfaces. *Progress in Experimental Tumour Research* **5**, 85.

Boutin, P. (1974) Les prothèses totales de la hanche en alumine. L'ancrage direct sans ciment dans 50 cas. *Revue de Chirurgie Orthopédique et Réparatrice de l'Appareil Moteur* **60**, 233.

Brånemark, P.-I., Lindström, J., Hallén, O., Breine, U., Jeppson, P. H. and Öhman, A. (1975) Reconstruction of the defective mandible. *Scandinavian Journal of Plastic and Reconstructive Surgery* **9**, 116.

Brendlinger, D. L. and Tarsitano, J. J. (1970) Generalized dermatitis due to sensitivity to a chrome cobalt removable partial denture. *Journal of the American Dental Association* **81**, 392.

Cameron, H., MacNab, I. and Pilliar, R. (1972) Porous surfaced vitallium staples. *South African Journal of Surgery* **10**, 63.

Cameron, H. U., Pilliar, R. M. and MacNab, I. (1973) The effect of movement on the bonding of porous metal to bone. *Journal of Biomedical Materials Research* **7**, 301.

Carter, R. L. and Roe, F. J. C. (1969) Induction of sarcomas in rats by solid and fragmented polyethylene: experimental observations and clinical implications. *British Journal of Cancer* **23**, 401.

Charnley, J. (1970) *Acrylic Cement in Orthopaedic Surgery*. Edinburgh and London, Churchill Livingstone.

Charosky, C. B., Bullough, P. G. and Wilson, P. D. Jr. (1973) Total hip replacement failures. A histological evaluation. *Journal of Bone and Joint Surgery* **55A**, 49.

Coleman, R. F., Herrington, J. and Scales, J. T. (1973) Concentration of wear products in hair, blood and urine after total hip replacement. *British Medical Journal* **1**, 527.

Elves, M. W., Wilson, J. N., Scales, J. T. and Kemp, H. B. S. (1975) Incidence of metal sensitivity in patients with total joint replacements. *British Medical Journal* **4**, 376.

Evans, E. M., Freeman, M. A. R., Miller, A. J. and Vernon-Roberts, B. (1974). Metal sensitivity as a cause of bone necrosis and loosening of the prosthesis in total joint replacement. *Journal of Bone and Joint Surgery* **56B**, 626.

Feith, R., Sloof, T. J. J. H., Kazem, I. and van Rens, T. J. G. (1976) Strontium ^{87m}Sr bone scanning for the evaluation of total hip replacement. *Journal of Bone and Joint Surgery* **58B**, 79.

Ferguson, A. B. Jr., Laing, P. G. and Hodge, E. S. (1960) The ionization of metal implants in living tissues. *Journal of Bone and Joint Surgery* **42A**, 77.

Freeman, M. A. R. (1975) General considerations in the design of prostheses for the 'total' replacement of joints. In, *Recent Advances in Orthopaedics*, No. 2, p. 93. Ed. B. McKibbin. Edinburgh and London, Churchill Livingstone.

Fregert, S. and Rorsman, H. (1966a) Allergic reactions to trivalent chromium compounds. *Archives of Dermatology* **93**, 711.

Fregert, S. and Rorsman, H. (1966b) Allergy to chromium, nickel and cobalt. *Acta Dermato-venereologica* **46**, 144.

Galante, J., Rostoker, W., Lueck, R. and Ray, D. (1971) Sintered fiber metal composites as a basis for attachment of implants to bone. *Journal of Bone and Joint Surgery* **53A**, 101.

Geduldig, D., Dörre, E., Happel, M., Lade, R., Prüssner, P., Willert, H.-G. and Zichner, L. (1975). Welche Aussicht hat die Biokeramik als Implantatmaterial in der Orthopädie? *Medizinisch-Orthopädische Technik* **6**, 138.

Griss, P., Krempien, B., von Andrian-Werburg, H., Heimke, G. and Fleiner, R. (1973) Experimentelle Untersuchung zur Gewebsverträglichkeit oxidkeramischer (Al_2O_3) Abriebteilchen. *Archiv für Orthopädische und Unfall-Chirurgie* **76**, 270.

Heath, J. C. and Daniel, M. R. (1962) The production of malignant tumours by cobalt in the rat: intrathoracic tumours. *British Journal of Cancer* **16**, 473.

Heath, J. C., Freeman, M. A. R. and Swanson, S. A. V. (1971) Carcinogenic properties of wear particles from prostheses made in cobalt chromium alloy. *Lancet* **1**, 564.

Homsy, C. A., Cain, T. E., Kessler, F. B., Anderson, S. and King, J. W. (1972) Porous implant systems for prosthesis stabilization. *Clinical Orthopaedics and Related Research* **89**, 220.

Howe, D. F., Svare, C. W. and Tock, R. W. (1975) Some effects of pore diameter on single pore bony ingression patterns in Teflon. *Journal of Biomedical Materials Research* **8**, 399.

Hulbert, S. F., Matthews, J. R., Klawitter, J. J., Sauer, B. W. and Leonard, R. B. (1974) Effect of stress on tissue ingrowth into porous aluminium oxide. *Journal of Biomedical Materials Research, Symposium No. 5*, part 1, p. 85.

Jefferiss, C. D., Lee, A. J. C. and Ling, R. S. M. (1975) Thermal aspects of self-curing polymethylmethacrylate. *Journal of Bone and Joint Surgery* **57B**, 511.

Jones, D. A., Lucas, H. K., O'Driscoll, M., Price, C. H. G. and Wibberley, B. (1975) Cobalt toxicity after McKee hip arthroplasty. *Journal of Bone and Joint Surgery* **57B**, 289.

Klawitter, J. J. and Hulbert, S. F. (1971) Application of porous ceramics for the attachment of load bearing internal orthopaedic applications. *Journal of Biomedical Materials Research, Symposium No. 2*, p. 161.

Klawitter, J. J., Bagwell, J. G., Weinstein, A. M. and Sauer, B. W. (1976) An evaluation of bone growth into porous high density polyethylene. *Journal of Biomedical Materials Research* **10**, 311.

Labitzke, R. and Paulus, M. (1974) Intraoperativ Temperaturmessungen in der Hüftchirurgie während der Polymerisation des Knochenzementes Palacos. *Archiv für Orthopädische und Unfall-Chirurgie* **79**, 341.

Laugier, P. and Foussereau, J. (1966) Les dermites allergiques à distance provoquées par le matériel d'osteosynthèse. *Gazette Médicale de France* **73**, 3409.

Lembert, E., Galante, J. and Rostoker, W. (1972) Fixation of skeletal replacement by fiber metal composites. *Clinical Orthopaedics and Related Research* **87**, 303.

Linder, L. and Lundskog, L. (1975) Incorporation of stainless steel, titanium and Vitallium in bone. *Injury* **6**, 277.

Lundskog, L. (1972) Heat and bone tissue. An experimental investigation of the thermal properties of bone and the threshold levels for thermal injury. *Scandinavian Journal of Plastic and Reconstructive Surgery* **9**, 1.

Lyng, S., Sudmann, E., Hulbert, S. F. and Sauer, B. W. (1973) Fixation of permanent orthopaedic prostheses. Use of ceramics in the tibial plateau. *Acta Orthopaedica Scandinavica* **44**, 694.

McKenzie, A. W., Aitken, C. V. E. and Risdill-Smith, R. (1967) Urticaria after insertion of Smith–Petersen Vitallium nail. *British Medical Journal* **4**, 36.

Mittelmeier, H. (1975) Selbsthaftende Keramik-Metall-Verbund-Endoprothesen. *Medizinisch-Orthopädische Technik* **95**, 152.

Mowat, A. G. and Hothersall, T. E. (1968) Nature of anaemia in rheumatoid arthritis—VIII. Iron content of synovial tissue in patients with rheumatoid arthritis and other joint diseases. *Annals of the Rheumatic Diseases* **27**, 345.

Muirden, K. D. and Senator, G. B. (1968) Iron in the synovial membrane in rheumatoid arthritis and other joint diseases. *Annals of the Rheumatic Diseases* **27**, 38.

Murray, W. R. and Rodrigo, J. J. (1975) Arthrography for the assessment of pain after total hip replacement. A comparison of arthrographic findings in patients with and without pain. *Journal of Bone and Joint Surgery* **57A**, 1060.

Nilles, J. L., Coletti, J. M. Jr. and Wilson C. (1973) Biomechanical evaluation of bone–porous material interfaces. *Journal of Biomedical Materials Research* **7**, 231.

Nothdurft, H. (1955) Über die Sarkomauslösung durch Fremdkörperimplantation bei Ratten in Abhängigkeit von der Form de Implantate. *Naturwissenschaften* **42**, 106.

Ohnsorge, J. and Goebel, G. (1970) Die Verwendung unterkühlter Metallendoprothesen in der Hüftchirurgie. *Zeitschrift für Orthopädie und ihre Grenzgebiete* **107**, 683.

Oppenheimer, B. S., Oppenheimer, E. T., Danishefsky, I, Stout, A. P. and Eirich, F. R. (1955) Further studies of polymers as carcinogenic agents in animals. *Cancer Research* **15**, 333.

Oppenheimer, B. S., Oppenheimer, E. T., Danishefsky, I. and Stout, A. P. (1956) Carcinogenic effect of metals in rodents. *Cancer Research* **16**, 439.

Oppenheimer, B. S., Oppenheimer, E. T., Stout, A. P., Danishefsky, I. and Willhite, M. (1959) Studies of the mechanism of carcinogenesis by plastic films. *Acta Unio Internationalis contra Cancrum* **15**, 659.

Oppenheimer, E. T., Willhite, M., Danishefsky, I. and Stout, A. P. (1961) Observations on the effect of powdered polymer in the carcinogenic process. *Cancer Research* **21**, 132.

Owen, R., Meachim, G. and Williams, D. F. (1976) Hair sampling for chromium content following Charnley hip arthroplasty. *Journal of Biomedical Materials Research* **10**, 91.

Rae, T. (1975) A study on the effects of particulate metals of orthopaedic interest on murine macrophages in vitro. *Journal of Bone and Joint Surgery* **57B**, 444.

Sauer, B. W., Klawitter, J. J., Weinstein, A. M. and Spector, M. (1976) The use of polymers in high load bearing joints in the locomotor system. In, *Engineering in Medicine*, Vol. 2. Berlin, Springer-Verlag.

Semlitsch, M., Vogel, A. and Willert, H.-G. (1972) Investigation of joint endoprostheses abrasion products in the connective tissue of the joint cavity. *Sulzer Technical Review* **2**, 137.

Swanson, S. A. V., Freeman, M. A. R. and Day, W. H. (1971) The fatigue properties of human cortical bone. *Medical and Biological Engineering* **9**, 23.

Swanson, S. A. V., Freeman, M. A. R. and Heath, J. C. (1973) Laboratory tests on total joint replacement prostheses. *Journal of Bone and Joint Surgery* **55B**, 759.

Szepesi, K. and Kapitany, S. (1974) Druckprobe zur Beurteilung der Tragfähigkeit des Femurkopfes in Tierversuchen. *Archiv für Orthopädische und Unfall-Chirurgie* **79**, 21.

Szepesi, K., Kapitany, S. and Csorba, E. (1974) Tragfähigkeit des Femurkopfes nach experimenteller ischämischer Nekrose der Epiphyse. II. Mechanische, röntgenologische Untersuchung und Untersuchung des Balkensystems. *Archiv für Orthopädische und Unfall-Chirurgie* **80**, 283.

Uhtoff, H. K. (1973) Mechanical factors influencing the holding power of screws in compact bone. *Journal of Bone and Joint Surgery* **55B**, 633.

Vernon-Roberts, B. and Freeman, M. A. R. (1976) Morphological and analytical studies of the tissues adjacent to joint prostheses: investigations into the causes of loosening of prostheses. In, *Engineering in Medicine*, Vol. 2. Berlin, Springer-Verlag.

Walker, P. S., Mendes, D. G., Figarola, F. and Bullough, P. G. (1974) Total surface replacement of the hip joint. In, *Prostheses and Tissue: the Interface Problem*, p. 245. Ed. S. F. Hulbert, S. N. Levine and D. D. Moyle. New York and Chichester, John Wiley.

Welsh, R. P., Pilliar, R. M. and MacNab, I. (1971) Surgical implants: the role of surface porosity in fixation to bone and acrylic. *Journal of Bone and Joint Surgery* **53A**, 963.

Willert, H.-G. (1973) Tissue reactions around joint implants and bone cement. In, *Arthroplasty of the Hip*, p. 11. Ed. G. Chapchal. Stuttgart, Thieme.

Willert, H.-G. and Puls, P. (1972) Die Reaktion des Knochens auf Knochenzement bei der Allo-Arthroplastik der Hüfte. *Archiv für Orthopädische und Unfall-Chirurgie* **72**, 33.

Willert, H.-G. and Semlitsch, M. (1974) Articular capsule reactions associated with joint endoprostheses. Congress of Dutch–Swiss Orthopaedic Societies, abstract published by Sulzer Brothers Ltd, Winterthur.

Willert, H.-G., Ludwig, J. and Semlitsch, M. (1974) Reaction of bone to methacrylate after hip arthroplasty. A long-term gross, light microscopic and scanning electron microscopic study. *Journal of Bone and Joint Surgery* **56A**, 1368.

Williams, D. F. (1973) The response of the body environment to implants. In, *Implants in Surgery*, p. 203. Ed. D. F. Williams and R. Roaf. Philadelphia, Pa., and London, W. B. Saunders.

Winter, G. D. (1974) Tissue reactions to metallic wear and corrosion products in human patients. *Journal of Biomedical Materials Research* **8**, 11.

CHAPTER FIVE

Mechanical Aspects of Fixation

1 INTRODUCTION

1.1 Acceptable Fixation

IT is required that the prosthetic components when subjected to repeated loads for periods measured in tens of years should not loosen sufficiently to give rise to pain or disability, that the patient should be able to move the joint concerned as soon as possible post-operatively, and that all foreign material should be removable if necessary.

This statement of requirements recognises firstly that there is no such thing as absolute rigidity. The bone to which the components are to be fixed is itself elastic, and deforms and recovers its shape under each application and removal of load. Since deformation occurs within the bone and since the prosthetic components also deform elastically, but to different extents because their materials have stiffnesses different from that of bone, some deformation at the bone–prosthesis interface seems inevitable and not necessarily harmful; the question is how much deformation is acceptable. The pragmatic answer is that on the macroscopic scale a cyclic displacement of the prosthetic component relative to the bone is acceptable if its magnitude does not progressively increase with repeated applications of load and if it does not give rise to pain or to the presence of unacceptable quantities of debris. What happens macroscopically will often result from what happens on the microscopic scale, and these events will be considered below. The statement of requirements recognises secondly that the fatigue strength of the interface, and not only its static strength, is relevant, and thirdly that the passage of time may lead to changes in the properties of the bone or of the other materials concerned.

1.2 Potentially Useful Methods of Fixation

From the purely mechanical point of view, several methods of fitting the prosthetic components to the bones could apparently be used. The obvious methods are:

> fitting the components directly to the bones, relying on interference between the gross shapes of the components and the bones;
> screwing, either by arranging a prosthetic component in the form of a screw or by using bone screws passing through holes in the component;
> the use of nuts and bolts;
> fitting the prosthetic components directly to the bones, relying not only on the gross shapes but also on interlock with designed surface features;
> using an adhesive;
> using a gap-filling agent ('cement') to fit the components to the bone;
> relying on the bone to grow into suitable holes or depressions in the surface of the component.

These methods have been listed in roughly the chronological order in which they have been tried in practice; two or more methods can sometimes be used together.

It would be possible to discuss each method in turn and to discuss the reasons for the success or failure of each. Since, however, clinical experience and laboratory observations now enable certain generalisations to be made about the biological response to endoprostheses and hence about the biological restrictions on any proposed mechanical solution to the problem of fixation, it is more efficient to consider these biological restrictions first and then to examine the mechanical possibilities in that light.

1.3 Biological Restrictions

Bone, both cortical and cancellous, is significantly weaker in static tension than in compression (Swanson 1971). Although experimental measurements have not been published, it is certain that the corresponding difference in fatigue is at least as great, and probably greater. If prosthetic components were bonded directly to bone, it would therefore be advisable to arrange that tensile stresses at the interface were, as far as possible, lower than compressive stresses.

In fact, few prosthetic components are bonded directly to bone after the initial phases of reaction by the host tissues. Histological observations made on specimens where acrylic cement had been used to fix prostheses (see Chapter 4; and Charnley 1970; Amstutz, Lurie and Bullough 1972; Willert and Puls 1972; Willert, Ludwig and Semlitsch 1974) and where a metallic prosthetic component has initially been in immediate contact with bone (Biehl, Harms and Mäusle 1975), all show that a layer of fibrous tissue is present at about a year after implantation. The origin, nature and thickness of this layer are discussed in Chapter 4; the present point is that such a layer is likely to be weak in tension and in shear, but reasonably durable in compression. It would therefore be wise to design prostheses and their attachments so as to avoid, if possible, tensile and shear stresses at the interfaces.

There is some evidence that bone will grow in apposition to certain ceramics without an intervening layer of fibrous tissue (Lyng et al. 1973; Hulbert et al. 1974). If this state were regularly achieved in clinical practice, the durability to be considered would be that of the bone and not that of a fibrous tissue layer; the resulting limitations would depend on the details of the bone–prosthesis interface, but would still include a lower limit on tensile than on compressive stresses. Thus a prosthesis designed to be secure with a fibrous layer present would still be safe, perhaps unnecessarily so, if such a layer were absent.

In summary, therefore, prostheses should be designed so that tensile and shear stresses at the interfaces are as small as possible, preferably zero, and compressive stresses are at a level that will not cause fatigue failure in the bone.

1.4 Effects of Biological Restrictions on Mechanical Design

Accepting the restrictions described above, the first question to be considered is how the stresses at the interface can be controlled to minimise tensile and shear stresses and limit compressive stresses. The types of force which can be transmitted to the interfaces depend on the shapes of the articulating surfaces, and these must therefore be considered. When the types of force which can be transmitted are known, the interfaces must then be designed to ensure, if possible, that these forces are transmitted across the interfaces as stresses of acceptable kinds and magnitudes.

Given that, as was shown in Chapter 2 and will be mentioned further below, it is in general not possible to arrange that the force at any one joint will always act in the same direction, the need for some geometrical interlock between the prosthetic component and the bone will become apparent. Some of the potentially useful methods listed above can then be considered in terms of their ability to provide the necessary interlock, both at the time of implantation and years later.

2 THE CONTROL OF INTERFACE STRESSES BY PROSTHETIC DESIGN

2.1 Design of the Articulating Surfaces

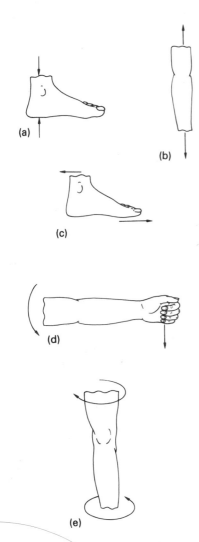

Figure 5.1.
Transmission of (a) compression, (b) tension, (c) shear, (d) bending, and (e) torsion loads by joints.

Theoretically, a joint, whether natural or prosthetic, could transmit loads of any of the following types: compression, tension, shear, bending, or torsion. These are illustrated in Fig. 5.1. Every joint in the body is subjected to compressive loading, and this may be regarded as the characteristic loading in normal use, to which the articular cartilage and subchondral bone are well adapted. Although tensile loads can be applied to limbs (by so ordinary a practice as carrying a case, as well as by gymnastics which are unlikely to concern patients with prosthetic joints), these are almost always transmitted across joints by muscles and ligaments and not by the joint surfaces; indeed, even when the limb as a whole is in tension, the joint surfaces may be in compression as a consequence of muscle action.

The three other forms of loading—shear, bending and torsion—can all arise in everyday activities and in minor accidents, and are usually transmitted through natural joints partly by compressive stresses between the articular surfaces and partly by tension in ligaments, because most natural joints are so shaped that only compressive (and sometimes torsion) loads can be transmitted by the former. Here may arise an important difference between natural and prosthetic joints: if the prosthetic joint replaces only the function of the articular surfaces, the loads transmitted across it will be compressive; but if it replaces also the function of the ligaments, it will transmit tensile and perhaps torsion loads as well as compressive loads with possibly undesirable consequences for the bone–prosthesis bond. However, if some or all of the ligaments have been damaged, a prosthesis which does not replace their function may be unstable or exposed to an increased risk of subluxation or dislocation.

Thus in the design of the articulating surfaces, a conflict arises: a prosthetic joint which replaces the ligaments and hence cannot sublux (or in the limit dislocate) is more likely to loosen, and one which minimises the risk of loosening by replacing only the articular surfaces and hence minimising the tensile forces at its attachments is likely to sublux. To such a design problem there is no unique solution, but it is clear that a prosthesis which loosens in response to repeated applications of normal loads is useless, as would be one which dislocated during everyday activities, and that the extremes of choice must therefore be avoided. Remembering that loosening implies the failure of that surgical treatment and perhaps a further operation, and that subluxation (especially if spontaneously reducible) is in general less serious, it seems reasonable to accept the risk of subluxation rather than loosening as a consequence of accidental overload; it also seems reasonable to accept, in everyday activities, repeated spontaneously reducing subluxations (which may be symptomless) if this is the price of freedom from loosening. Two pairs of

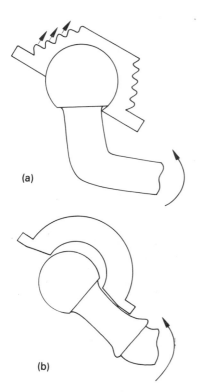

(a)

(b)

examples can be given. At the hip, a cup which is no more than hemispherical will allow subluxation (during, perhaps, hyperadduction or squatting). There is little doubt that this happens, unnoticed, in many patients and that it is greatly preferable to the increased risk of loosening which would be present with a femoral head positively retained in a more than hemispherical cup, a feature which is incorporated in some designs to eliminate the possibility of dislocation. At the knee, a fully constrained hinge cannot sublux or dislocate but imposes on its attachments bending loads with the attendant risks of loosening, whereas the many types of unlinked surface replacement prostheses are much less likely to impose tensile forces on their attachments but can, and probably do, sublux repeatedly in everyday activities. These comparisons are illustrated in Fig. 5.2.

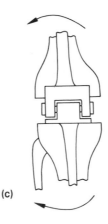

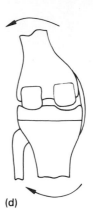

(c)

(d)

Figure 5.2.
(a) Hip prosthesis with more-than-hemispherical cup, not free to sublux, transmitting tensile forces to the interface. (b) Hip prosthesis free to sublux. (c) Hinged knee prosthesis, transmitting bending loads to the interfaces when loaded in abduction. (d) Unlinked surface replacement knee prosthesis, free to sublux but unable to transmit tensile forces to the interfaces.

Such 'subluxation' is harmless in itself, being similar to that which is possible in a natural knee (in which the condyles can be separated by abduction or adduction of the tibia) but the possibility should not be overlooked that if it occurs under even moderate loads, locally high stresses may accelerate the wear of the articulating surfaces.

Even with a prosthesis which is free to sublux, some shear and tensile forces may in certain circumstances be transmitted to the interfaces. For example, if as in Fig. 5.3 forces are applied to a leg tending to sublux the tibia anteriorly on the femur, some shear force

Figure 5.3.
Transmission of shear force across an unlinked surface replacement knee prosthesis.

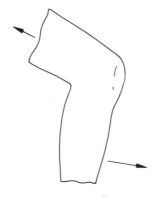

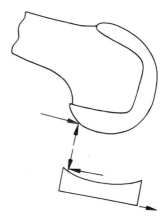

will be transmitted across the articulating surfaces of even an unlinked surface replacement type of prosthesis. The magnitude of the transmitted shear force will depend on the shapes of the articulating surfaces, the coefficient of friction between them, and the compressive force keeping them together, but in practice it is most unlikely to be zero.

If the articulating surfaces are designed to replace only the functions of the natural articular surfaces and not those of the ligaments, they cannot transmit resultant forces which are tensile; but a compressive or shear force can be applied in such a way as to give rise to tensile forces at some part of the interface. Figure 5.4 shows a force applied anteriorly by the femoral component to the tibial component of an unlinked surface replacement knee prosthesis. If the tibial component has been implanted so as not to engage the anterior cortex of the tibia, or if it rests partly on a region of porotic bone or a cyst, there will be a tendency for it to 'rock' about a fulcrum of relatively stiff bone, as indicated in Fig. 5.4. Then the only way to prevent the prosthetic component coming loose is for tensile forces to be exerted on its posterior part in a downward direction.

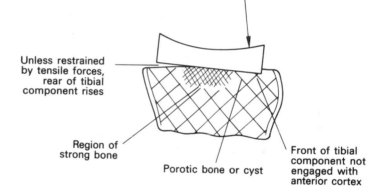

Figure 5.4.
Irregular support to the tibial component of a knee prosthesis, leading to 'rocking' and the need for tensile forces to preserve equilibrium.

Unless restrained by tensile forces, rear of tibial component rises

Region of strong bone

Porotic bone or cyst

Front of tibial component not engaged with anterior cortex

In the above discussion, tensile forces at the prosthesis–bone interface have been introduced in the sense that in certain circumstances the equilibrium of a prosthetic component requires that these forces exist. As has been accepted for the purpose of the present discussion, few real interfaces can transmit significant tensile forces, and this means that in some circumstances equilibrium will not be preserved; i.e. the prosthetic component will loosen.

To summarise, if the articulating surfaces of prostheses are so shaped that they do not replace the functions of the ligaments and are in consequence able to sublux, the transmission of tensile and shear forces to the bone–prosthesis interfaces will be minimised but not eliminated, and the forces at these interfaces will therefore be predominantly, but not exclusively, compressive in nature.

2.2 Design of the Prosthesis–Bone Interface

Given that compressive forces at the interface are inevitable, and that by attention to the design of the articulating surfaces tensile and shear forces at the interface can be reduced, but not to zero, the question arises of designing the interface to keep all the corresponding stresses to acceptable levels.

The stress corresponding to a given compressive force is reduced by increasing the area of interface perpendicular to that force. For this purpose, the projected area of an inclined interface is as effective as the area of an interface at right angles to the force (Fig. 5.5), but area parallel to the direction of the force is irrelevant. Thus, if only compressive loads acting in one direction had to be transmitted, a flat surface on the femoral component of a knee or hip prosthesis would be just as effective as the projected area of a tapered stem. Even when the articulating surfaces have been designed to restrict the transmission of forces, in ways discussed above, at almost any joint forces must be expected to act at some times in different directions, and therefore the provision of a large area facing in one direction is not sufficient in a real joint; but whatever more elaborate arrangements are made must include sufficient area in the relevant directions.

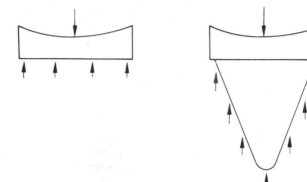

Figure 5.5.
The equivalence of the area of an inclined interface to that of one at right angles to the applied force.

The desirable level of compressive stress must be specified on an empirical basis. If it is too high, there is a danger of fatigue failure in the bone; but little is known of the fatigue properties of cortical bone and nothing about those of cancellous bone. Observation shows that some prostheses do sink into the cancellous bone supporting them, and this suggests that in practice the margin of safety is non-existent in some patients and therefore probably not very large in any patient. This in turn suggests that the general aim should be to reduce compressive stresses as much as possible by providing the biggest practicable area of interface perpendicular to the applied forces. (There is a theoretical danger of reducing the stresses so far as to introduce the danger of disuse-osteoporosis. This is most unlikely to arise with surface replacement types of prosthesis, because at a short distance from the prosthesis the whole of the available bone is transmitting loads much as it would in a natural joint. Arrangements which depart further from the natural (for example, by introducing a rigid intramedullary stem which will transmit a large fraction of the load that would otherwise have been transmitted by the bone) may, however, raise the danger of localised disuse-osteoporosis in practice as well as in theory.) In general it is desirable to engage the whole of the cross-section which is available, including particularly the cortical bone which is stronger statically, and presumably also in fatigue, than the same cross-sectional area of cancellous bone. At any level, as with any contact between two solids, the effective area of contact is a small fraction of the apparent area because only the high points on the two surfaces touch. Therefore any agent such as cement, which can increase the effective area of contact, will decrease the general level of stress.

Still considering the stresses on small elements of an interface (as distinct from forces on a whole interface), most forms of interface cannot transmit tensile stresses, and those which can (conceivably, a rough surface cemented to a cancellous bone, and, more probably, a porous surface with bone ingrowth) are still subject to the limitation that bone is weaker in tension than in compression. Therefore the chief consideration must be not merely how to reduce tensile stresses to the same level as compressive stresses, but how to eliminate them.

Tensile stresses can be replaced by compressive stresses if an interlocking interface is provided. Figure 5.6 shows a simple example in which compressive forces are transmitted as compressive stresses acting on the lower surfaces of the projecting rings on the implant, and tensile forces as compressive stresses acting on the upper surfaces of the rings. Shear stresses will act on the surfaces parallel to the load axis, unless the interface has no shear strength. Such an arrangement can remain firmly fixed even if the tensile strength of the interfaces is zero; only the tolerance of the materials to compressive (and perhaps shear) stress is involved.

The problems of achieving such interlocking are considered below; here it is sufficient to note that some interlocking can be achieved at all joints, but not usually so effectively as to eliminate the need to reduce tensile forces by attention to the shapes of the articulating surfaces.

2.2.2 TENSILE STRESSES

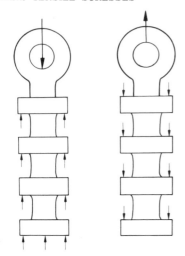

Figure 5.6.
A simple interlocking interface which transmits either tensile or compressive forces as compressive stresses.

2.2.3 SHEAR STRESSES

These usually act when shear or torsional loads are applied, but can also be the means of transmitting tensile or compressive loads. Figure 5.7a shows a tibial plateau subjected to torsion; if the interface with the bone is completely flat, all the torsion is transmitted by shear stresses at the interface. Figure 5.7b shows a tibial component with no horizontal flange and a parallel-sided intramedullary stem; in this improbable arrangement, compressive forces would be transmitted entirely by shear stresses acting longitudinally at the interface. If, as in Fig. 5.7c, a flange is provided and the intramedullary interface is tapered, compressive forces are transmitted partly

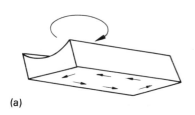

(a)

Figure 5.7.
(a) Torsion applied to a tibial plateau and transmitted as shear stresses on a flat interface. (b) Compression applied to an unflanged tibial component and transmitted as shear stresses on the intramedullary stem. (c) Compression applied to a flanged tibial component and transmitted partly as compressive stresses applied to the flange, partly as compressive stresses on the tapered intramedullary stem, and partly as shear stresses on the stem.

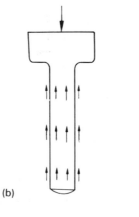

(b)

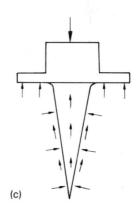

(c)

by compressive stresses on the flange, partly by compressive stresses on the medullary interface (because this interface, being tapered, has a component area perpendicular to the direction of the force), and partly by shear stresses on the medullary interface. (The term 'medullary interface' has been used here because for the present purpose it does not matter whether the implant is cemented in place or not; if it is, everything said about stresses applies both to the implant–cement surface and to the cement–bone interface if this is fairly smooth.) Whether the stem is tapered or parallel-sided, torsion applied to the prosthesis is transmitted partly by shear stresses acting on the flange, if any, and partly (in practice almost entirely, if the flange is smooth-surfaced) by shear stresses acting tangentially at the surface of the stem.

Clearly, neither bone nor cement will transmit significant shear stresses to a smooth surface, and surfaces of prostheses are therefore in practice equipped with projections which engage with either cement cured *in situ* or recesses in the bone. The effect of such projections is to replace shear stresses with compressive stresses, as shown in Fig. 5.8a. Similarly, intramedullary stems are given cross-sections having projections which transmit torsional loads (to bone or, more usually, cement) by compressive stresses, as indicated in Fig. 5.8b. Although cement is discussed below, it may be noted here that the same considerations apply to the cement–bone interface as to the prosthesis–bone interface; in a medullary canal of smooth circular cross-section, torsion would be transmitted from cement to bone as shear stresses, whereas with a non-circular cross-section the torsion is transmitted partly as compressive stresses.

From considerations of stress analysis (discussed in Chapter 2) it will be clear that, for a given torque to be transmitted, the shear and compressive stresses will be smaller if they can act at larger radii from the axis of the torque. Thus large projections, or several small projections widely spaced, will give low stresses, but obviously there may be practical limitations.

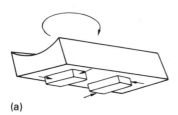

(a)

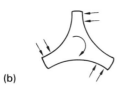

(b)

Figure 5.8.
Torsion applied to (a) a tibial plateau, and (b) an intramedullary stem and transmitted as compressive stresses on projections at the interface.

2.2.4 SUMMARY AND IMPLICATIONS

Compressive stresses arising from compressive forces can be minimised by providing the largest practicable area of interface perpendicular to the compressive forces to be transmitted. Tensile stresses cannot be developed beyond the tensile strength of the material, but the need for them can be eliminated by providing interlocking interfaces which will transmit tensile forces as compressive instead of tensile stresses. Shear stresses arising from torsional forces can largely be replaced with compressive stresses by providing suitably interlocking interfaces. Since all but the simplest forms of interface contain surfaces aligned in different directions, all forms of loading will be transmitted in part by shear stresses if the interface has any significant shear strength.

It is thus necessary to consider how to provide interfaces which will give the necessary interlocking both at the time of implantation and for years afterwards. If any particular method seems likely to offer good interlocking and fixation several months and longer after implantation, but cannot do so for the first few months, the question arises of arranging temporary support for those few months; one example of such a method is the growth of bone into rough-surfaced implants. It is therefore necessary, in examining each possible method, to consider not only whether it can provide the interlocking shown above to be desirable or necessary, but also whether it can do this at short times after implantation of the prosthesis, long times, or both.

3 TYPES OF INTERFACE

3.1 Adhesives

Adhesives are mentioned only to be dismissed as impracticable for the foreseeable future. If an adhesive is ever discovered which will adhere to metal or plastic and to bone in the conditions of surgery, and will continue to adhere to bone while the constituents of bone are turned over and loads are repeatedly applied, all while producing no harmful effects in the host tissues, it will be very attractive. No adhesive has so far been shown to have this combination of properties, and it seems unlikely that one will be.

3.2 Interference Fit of Implant

By this is meant a fit similar to that of a nail in wood; part of the implant occupies a hole in the bone which is too small for it, and elastic forces therefore ensure a frictional grip between the implant and the bone. (In joint replacement surgery as against carpentry, the hole is unlikely to be made by the driving in of the implant itself, because of the considerable risk of splitting the bone.) A simple example is the unfenestrated stem of a Thompson femoral head prosthesis impacted without cement into a reamed femoral canal.

An interference fit can be successful with wood or metals, but with living bone it suffers from the obvious limitation that remodelling of the bone can remove the interference on which the fixation depends. Invariably to attain an interference fit requires a precision of cutting bone which is unlikely to be practicable in routine practice in hospitals of varying types, and any movement of the prosthetic component relative to the bone is likely to lead to bone resorption and hence to increased loosening.

Thus interference fits cannot be regarded as suitable for permanent fixation in widespread practice, but may be suitable for the temporary fixation of implants whose long-term fixation depends on the growth of bone into recesses on the surface, as discussed below.

3.3 Components Attached with Separate Screws

3.3.1 SCREWS LOADED IN SHEAR

In theory, many load-bearing implants could be attached to bone by screws passing through the cortex of the shaft of a bone and through holes in an intramedullary stem, as indicated in Fig. 5.9a. This would not in itself ensure tightness of the stem in the medullary cavity, which would require either a precision of fit similar to that required for an interference fit as discussed above or a number of screws passing through holes made in different directions. The latter arrangement would involve extensive and probably unacceptable interference with the periosteum and increased operative complexity. Either arrangement would presumably give some incidence of the troubles, such as loosening of screws or crevice corrosion under the screwheads, encountered with fracture fixation devices embodying screws loaded in shear when delayed union or non-union prolongs the time for which they are needed. These troubles would be expected to occur months after implantation, and this suggests that the use of screws loaded in shear might be suitable only for temporary fixation, as was suggested above for interference fits.

3.3.2 SCREWS LOADED IN TENSION

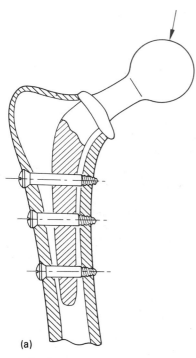

(a)

Figure 5.9.
(a) A femoral component of a hip prosthesis, fixed by screws which are loaded in shear. (b) The glenoid component of a shoulder prosthesis attached by screws, at least one of which is loaded in tension when a vertical load is transmitted through the joint. (c) The tibial component of a knee prosthesis attached by screws, the tension in which is reduced by the application of a vertical compressive force to the articulating surface.

Tensile loads on screws can arise from different causes. Whatever the shape of the component and the forces applied to it in service, when no external forces are applied to it any screws passing through it into the bone will be in tension if they have been driven in tightly. The application of external forces may either increase or decrease these loads built in during implantation. For example, if the glenoid component of a fully constrained ball-and-socket shoulder prosthesis is attached with screws, vertical or anteroposterior forces applied to the joint will produce increased tension in at least one screw, as shown in Fig. 5.9b. If, in contrast, the tibial component of a surface replacement type of knee prosthesis were to be attached to the tibia using vertical screws, as in Fig. 5.9c, the effect of a vertical compressive force would be to compress the component and the underlying bone, and even an elastic compression would probably be sufficient to reduce the tensile force in the screws, conceivably to zero. A similar arrangement could be used at the acetabulum, using screws passing through holes in a flange round the rim of the cup, the axes of the screws thus being nearly parallel to the line of action of the highest load on the joint.

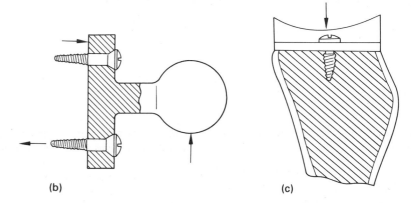

(b)

(c)

In any such arrangement, the same reservations must apply as were mentioned above about the long-term strength of screws in bone, particularly where the location of the prosthetic component depends entirely on the tensile strength of one or two screws in bone, as in the glenoid component chosen as an example. With the tibial or acetabular components, most or all of the compressive load would be transmitted to the bone by the surface of the prosthetic component in contact with it, the screws being largely redundant for this purpose. Then problems of locally high contact pressures, resorption and loosening would be expected to arise almost as if the screws were not present. These problems could be alleviated by some other means, but the screws alone could not alleviate them.

3.3.3 CONCLUSIONS

The theoretical considerations advanced above, and the clinical incidence of loosening and corrosion with screwed fracture fixation devices, give no ground for confidence that screws alone, whatever the nature of the loads on the screws, would give reliable long-term fixation, although they may be suitable for the temporary fixation of an implant while bone growth into a suitable surface establishes the permanent fixation.

3.4 Components Attached with Nuts and Bolts

The limitations of this method are similar to those surrounding the use of screws. In many prostheses it would simply not be possible to arrange for a nut and bolt to be used, and in others where it would be possible it would be undesirable to incur the extra exposure and interference with the periosteum. Nuts and bolts cannot therefore be regarded as a method worth serious consideration for general application.

3.5 Cement

By 'cement' is meant a substance which is cast *in situ* to fill the gap between a prosthetic component and the bone. With this definition, adhesion of the cement to the prosthetic component, the bone, or both, is a bonus; what matters is that it should set with an accurate fit to both surfaces. The only cement so far widely used is, of course, methyl methacrylate polymerised *in situ*, and all thinking about this aspect of fixation has been conditioned by the properties of this particular cement; but it is unlikely that any cement which might replace it in the foreseeable future would have radically different mechanical properties. The present discussion is concerned with cement as a means of providing interlocking; certain mechanical properties of polymethylmethacrylate and other possible cements are considered later in this chapter, while biological aspects of the use of polymethylmethacrylate were considered in Chapter 4.

It is generally recognised that the cement fits the inner surface of the bone and the outer surface of the prosthetic component as closely as possible. It may adhere to the surface of the prosthetic component, if this is clean and dry, but the adhesion will have limited strength; little or no adhesion takes place between the cement and the bone, which is usually wet and greasy. Thus the mechanical effect of cement is to distribute load over the largest possible contact area and so to give the lowest possible contact stresses. If mechanical interlocking takes place (assisted by suitable preparation of the bony bed), freedom from loosening under ordinary loads is virtually guaranteed for as long as the interlocking lasts. Apart from violence, the interlocking could, in principle, be removed by infection or by the short-term or long-term adjustment of the tissues following the introduction of the cement. A number of histological observations have been made on uninfected and clinically satisfactory specimens, at times up to several years after implantation. These observations, reviewed in Chapter 4, show that about two years after implantation the acrylic cement is separated from the bone or marrow tissue by a layer of fibrous tissue.

If these observations, few in number, are representative, it seems that one must expect continuous remodelling to increase the smoothness of the bone surface, leaving the irregular gap between that and the cement surface to be filled by soft tissue. If this were to happen (and whether or not it will happen after 10 or 20 years of implantation is not yet known), the long-term security of fixation with cement would be similar to that of direct fixation. It follows that provision must be made for interlocking into bone at a size of several millimetres. Whether this is done by providing projections on the prosthetic components and surrounding them with a thin layer of cement, or by making suitable recesses in the bone and filling these with cement, is a secondary matter. Figure 5.10 indicates the two possibilities. Whichever form is used, the interlock with the bone

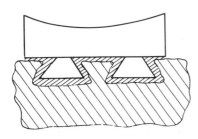

(a)

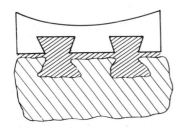

(b)

Figure 5.10.
Interlock with bone provided (a) by projections on the prosthetic component surrounded by a thin layer of cement, and (b) by cement filling a recess in the bone.

will be maintained even if bone is replaced by fibrous tissue to the extent so far observed; fibrous replacement of bone on a scale not yet observed would be needed to remove the interlock.

To take a simple example of the absence of such interlock, if an intramedullary stem is cemented into a medullary cavity which is essentially conical in shape and circular in cross-section, the early postoperative fixation is likely to be good if the endosteal surface was rough but firm; but in a few years the cement–bone interface will consist of a conical sheet of fibrous tissue, with little or no microscopic interdigitation of bone and cement. The resistance of this interface to compression would depend partly on the shear strength and partly on the compressive strength of the fibrous tissue, and would probably be sufficient (whether it was so would depend on the angle of the cone), but its resistance to torsion would depend entirely on the shear strength of the fibrous tissue, and might well be insufficient. This is an extreme example (though potentially a common one), but it illustrates the thesis that the bony interfaces should be so shaped as to provide sufficient interlocking to transmit loads at safe stresses.

Although cement cannot make a basically inadequate interlock adequate, it can, given a basically adequate interlock, enable an acceptable fixation to be routinely achieved with an accuracy of bone cutting which is likely to be practicable, whereas fixation without cement, as mentioned above, requires considerable and probably unrealistic accuracy. This repeatability is probably the most important result of the present widespread use of cement.

3.6 Interlock Provided by the Gross Shape of the Implant

3.6.1 NEED FOR INTERLOCK

In section 2.2, above, it was shown that some interlock is needed at the prosthesis–bone interface in order to ensure that forces applied to the prosthesis are transmitted across the interface mainly as compressive stresses and, to an acceptable extent, as shear stresses. Interference fits and screws have been dismissed as unlikely to provide secure fixation at long times after implantation. Cement will not in practice adhere to prosthetic components so as to give a useful strength. It is therefore necessary to consider how suitable interlocking can be provided by the shaping of the surfaces of the prosthetic components.

3.6.2 INTERLOCKING TO TRANSMIT COMPRESSION OR TENSION

The essential feature of interlocking which will transmit compressive or tensile forces as compressive stresses is the presence of projections (or depressions) which present an area perpendicular to the direction of the force to be transmitted, as shown in Fig. 5.6, above. This is simple in principle, but in practice the difficulty is encountered that most, if not all, prosthetic components must, for surgical reasons, be introduced in roughly the direction of the forces which will later be applied; all intramedullary stems come into this category. Obviously, the introduction of a prosthetic component in this way will ensure that the grooves or other formations on its surface are occupied by bone which has been sheared off the endosteal surface rather than by living bone contiguous with the host tissue. The ability of such an interface to transmit load for the first few months after implantation must therefore be seriously in doubt.

If such an implant could be inserted sideways into a prepared bony bed, this major deficiency would be circumvented, but clearly this is rarely, if ever, possible. If the grooves are formed on the surface of a tapered body, as on the acetabular component of the Sivash hip (Sivash 1969), or on the femoral component of a hip prosthesis as designed by Mittelmeier (1974), each groove can be occupied at least partly by firm bone at the time of implantation, and compressive loads can therefore be transmitted by compressive stresses; but the interlocking provides no resistance to tensile forces (which are unlikely to arise in hip prostheses, except for the curious circumstance that the Sivash hip is one of the few in which the femoral head is held captive in the acetabular component).

The only practicable way to provide transverse grooves which can be effective in tension or compression from the time of implantation of a prosthesis loaded in the direction in which it is inserted is to make them in the form of a screw thread on the outside of a body of circular cross-section. One example of this is the acetabular component of the Ring hip (Ring 1968), in which the cup is formed integrally with a screw about 75 mm long and 9 mm in diameter. Some acetabular cups (Griss, Heimke and Andrian-Werburg 1975) have cylindrical outer surfaces with circumferential grooves, and in one version (so far implanted only in sheep) these grooves are made in the form of a screw thread and the component is screwed into a prepared recess. The possibility must be considered that the cyclic variation in the magnitude and direction of the forces on the hip joint might tend to tighten the acetabular component on one side and to unscrew that on the other side. If this were shown to be a significant problem, components could be made with left- and right-handed screws.

3.6.3 INTERLOCKING TO TRANSMIT SHEAR OR TORSION

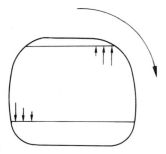

Figure 5.11.
View along the femoral shaft of the femoral component of a surface replacement type of knee prosthesis, showing how torsional loads are transmitted as compressive stresses at the interface.

The principles were outlined in section 2.2 and illustrated in Fig. 5.8 above, so far as they relate to the transmission of torsion by compressive stresses at the interface. In designing any interface to transmit torsion, it must be remembered that the stresses on the projections (or recesses) are reduced by placing the projections as far out from the axis of torsion as possible. In the femoral components of surface replacement knee prostheses for example, this is naturally and easily achieved by trimming the femoral condyles to the smallest possible extent and making the prosthetic component of a generally U shape. Figure 5.11 shows how torsion is transmitted by compressive stresses distributed across the contact surfaces, and it is obvious that smaller stresses are required if they act further from the axis of torsion. With other components, surgical or anatomical factors preclude so simple a solution and, instead of the shape of the component itself sufficing, projections have to be arranged on an otherwise unsuitably flat surface, as in the knee tibial component shown in Fig. 5.8a. The same principle holds, and compressive stresses are made low either by using several projections spaced as widely as practicable or by using one projection which is as big, mediolaterally and antero-posteriorly, as practicable. The thickness of the projection measured along the axis of torsion is also obviously relevant; its dimensions in all three directions are finally a compromise between conflicting aims: for example, if the projection is made too thick, there may be little cancellous bone for the distal part of it or its surrounding cement to interlock with, and the extra removal of cancellous bone will jeopardise an arthrodesis if this should ever be required. Similar considerations apply to prosthetic inserts for the bearing surface of the patella, and to the talar components of ankle prostheses. In all these joints the effectiveness of interlocking is limited by anatomical or surgical factors, and freedom from loosening therefore requires attention to the loads which can be transmitted by the articular surfaces of the prosthetic components, as discussed in section 2.1 above.

An interlocking interface which will transmit torsional loads as compressive stresses will almost certainly also transmit shear forces as compressive stresses. Consideration of the interfaces shown in Figs. 5.8a and 5.11 will show that some area is presented in directions perpendicular to the anteroposterior shear forces. Whether this area is large enough to keep the resulting compressive stresses to an acceptably low level depends, of course, on the ability of the articulating surfaces to transmit such shear forces; the interfaces and articulating surfaces cannot be rationally designed in isolation from each other. Areas on which compressive stress can act so as to transmit mediolateral shear forces can also be provided as in Fig. 5.8a.

3.6.4 PRACTICAL APPLICATION

It was suggested above, in section 3.5, that the use of cement alone (without suitable shaping of the prosthetic surface), the bony surface, or both, could not provide the interlocking which the considerations in section 2.2 showed to be necessary if load transmission across the interface is to be primarily by compressive stresses. It has now been shown that prosthetic components can be designed to present interfaces which will transmit as compressive stresses most or all of the loads which can be applied to them (assuming that the interfaces and articulating surfaces are designed together), but that surgical limitations on the ways in which components can be introduced at operation mean that some interlocking interfaces cannot be effective until sufficient time has elapsed for bone to grow into the surface features in question. In this circumstance, there are three possibilities: (1) a prolonged period of severely restricted load-bearing; (2) the provision of temporary support; or (3) the use of a gap-filling agent to make it unnecessary to wait for bone to grow into the interlocking surface features. Of these three, the third is the most attractive, at least if repeatedly good early results are sought, and is found in the widespread use of acrylic cement.

The point of the present discussion is to show that the provision of interlock by means of the gross shape of the implant, and the use of a cement, are complementary and equally necessary features of a system which will give good fixation at both short and long times after implantation.

3.7 Bone Ingrowth

3.7.1 INTRODUCTION

The problem of achieving interlocking could apparently be solved if the prosthetic component could be held in place for long enough to allow bone to grow into suitable recesses on the implant surface. These recesses could be many and small (less than a millimetre wide), amounting in effect to a rough or porous surface, or they could be fewer and larger (several millimetres wide), as the grooves round the outer surfaces of some acetabular cups (Boutin 1972, 1974; Griss, Heimke and Andrian-Werburg 1975). If ingrowth could be achieved, the difficulty, mentioned in section 3.6.2 above, that the grooves contain no useful bone because they shear it off as the component is inserted, would be circumvented.

The fenestrated stem of the Moore femoral head prosthesis could be regarded as the earliest example of this approach to fixation, but is obviously of limited application because the holes are too large to be effectively filled by bone. Work intended to lead to more widely useful techniques has been performed principally in the United States of America, perhaps with the incentive of the difficulty in that country of legalising the general use of any implant material which has not been fully tested; a porous-surfaced implant can offer the advantage of not introducing a material additional to that of the bulk implant, which presumably has been tested clinically.

The factors which influence the growth of bone into holes in a foreign body are largely biological, and have been considered in Chapter 4; the present discussion is concerned with the mechanical aspects.

3.7.2 MECHANICAL CONDITIONS FOR INGROWTH

In addition to the requirements of a biological nature (suitable material, viable bone, pore size in an acceptable range, etc.), there is a mechanical requirement that relative movement between the implant and the bone must be restricted during the weeks or months during which ingrowth is taking place. It is obvious that gross movement, an order of magnitude greater than the pore size, will prevent ingrowth, and this was confirmed by experiments reported by Cameron, Pilliar and MacNab (1973). Lyng et al. (1973) implanted ceramic pellets in the tibial plateau of dogs in such a way that the upper end of the cylindrical pellet protruded above the cartilage and was therefore cyclically loaded by the femoral condyle. The pellets were firmly anchored after six and eight weeks, bone and fibrous ingrowth being found in the pores the sizes of which were in the range 100–750 μm. Lembert, Galante and Rostoker (1972) found massive bone ingrowth into the porous-surfaced intramedullary stems of femoral head prostheses implanted into dogs which walked freely from the time of implantation. The porous surfaces were made of sintered titanium wire, giving a pore size of about 230 μm. These last two sets of observations are compatible with the idea that bone will grow into pores in a surface if, during the period of growth, the cyclic relative movement at the surface is less than the pore size. Presumably for substantial ingrowth the movement should be an order of magnitude less than the pore width, so that most of the width could be occupied by bone. Fibrous tissue presumably appears where cyclic movement interferes with the deposition of bone, and it would be interesting to see the results of a series of tests in which different and known cyclic movements were imposed while bone was growing into pores of standard size. Taking the minimum pore width for reliable ingrowth, without load on the implant, as 100 μm (on the basis of results reviewed in Chapter 4), a permissible relative movement of about 10 μm seems possible. Simple calculations, based on Young's moduli for compact bone and for implant alloys, show that the cyclic movement of parts of an intramedullary stem in a hip joint, loaded to three times body weight and adequately supported at the proximal end, should be about 10 μm. The comparison of the figures suggests that if temporary fixation can be achieved (by, for example, an interference fit), the intrinsic stiffnesses of the materials are such that bone could be expected to grow into holes in the surface of the implant.

It is obviously of interest to compare the strength of the bond between bone and a porous implant with that achieved using acrylic cement. Unfortunately, direct comparisons have been made only with porous-surfaced implanted plugs which had not been loaded. The results of such comparisons have usually been expressed as the shear strength calculated from the nominal surface area of the cylindrical interface and the force required to push the plug out of the bone when applied along the axis of the plug (which was sometimes perpendicular and sometimes parallel to the long axis of the bone). Such tests, on non-weight-bearing implants, may be taken to show the best performance that might be hoped for. Table 5.1 summarises results published by three groups in five papers.

Table 5.1   Shear Strengths of Bone–Porous Plug Interfaces*

Material	Source			
	Nilles, Coletti and Wilson (1973)	Welsh, Pilliar and MacNab (1971)	Cameron, Pilliar and MacNab (1973)	Galante et al. (1971) Lembert, Galante and Rostoker (1972)
Methyl methacrylate	2·0			1·5
Stainless steel (smooth)	1·5			
Stainless steel (porous)	15·0			
Ceramic (porous)	9·0	0·8–1·1		
Bone	25·0			
Co–Cr–Mo (sintered)		10.7–12·5	17	
Titanium (sintered)				1·4–2·4

* All strengths given in MN/m².

Nilles, Coletti and Wilson (1973) used plugs placed transversely in the cortices of long bones and tested them at times after implantation which histology showed to have given full ingrowth. For comparison, they included smooth-surfaced stainless steel, methyl methacrylate cured *in situ*, and bone which had grown into an otherwise unfilled hole of the same size as the plugs. Welsh, Pilliar and MacNab (1971) tested sintered Co–Cr–Mo alloy. Cameron, Pilliar and MacNab (1973) tested their static porous-surfaced Co–Cr–Mo staples. Galante et al. (1971) and Lembert, Galante and Rostoker (1972) tested plugs with sintered titanium surfaces impacted into slightly undersized holes in the medullary canal, and compared them with methyl methacrylate cured *in situ* and tested six weeks after implantation.

No definite conclusion can be drawn from these results, but it appears that if a porous-surfaced implant can be immobilised sufficiently to permit bone ingrowth, shear strengths at least equal to and probably greater than those obtained with methyl methacrylate can be expected.

The strength of the bond with a porous-surfaced implant may increase with time and then remain constant, whereas the strength of the bond with cement seems more likely to decrease with time.

Four important questions have not yet been fully answered: (1) how a load-bearing implant is to be held in place for several months while bone grows into the recesses on the surface; (2) whether bone which grows into recesses under little or no cyclic load will be replaced by fibrous tissue after a few years of cyclic loading; (3) whether the fatigue and corrosion behaviour of the implant material will be seriously affected by the presence of the corners and/or crevices in the porous layer; and (4) how an implant is to be removed. The first question is potentially soluble, since uncemented load-bearing implants do achieve secure fixation, and suitable design and careful operative technique could give enough security to allow restricted weight-bearing for the necessary few months. It may be doubted whether this could be achieved routinely at all joints and in all hospitals. In this connection, a fragile or readily deformable porous layer on the surface of a component seems more likely to lead to difficulties than a robust surface layer if interference fits have to be used. The second question can only be answered by extended clinical experience, but the observation of a fibrous layer partly filling serrations about 1 mm deep on the surface of an intramedullary stem one year after implantation of the hip prosthesis (Biehl, Harms and Mäusle 1975) is not encouraging. The answer to the third question also requires clinical experience, because laboratory tests could hardly reproduce the stress distributions consequent on the state of bone ingrowth after months or years. The fourth question is also potentially soluble in some circumstances. An infected implant would presumably not have been penetrated effectively by bone, so removal would not present a severe problem. A broken implant, particularly if the break were in an intramedullary stem, would present a worse problem than a broken cemented intramedullary stem. The need to replace worn prostheses could, in principle, be avoided by arranging for the wearing parts to be replaceable without disturbing the bulk implant, but this would be difficult in practice with prostheses consisting essentially of a surface shell.

Prostheses fixed by bone ingrowth may thus be found suitable for only certain kinds of joint; for example, those not requiring a long intramedullary stem and those which are unlikely to wear out or which could easily be made with a replaceable bearing surface.

3.8 Direct Chemical Bonding

If implants could be made having surfaces with which bone would form bonds which were chemical rather than mechanical, a more permanent fixation might be achieved than with any method relying on mechanical interlocking. Work by Hench and colleagues (Hench et al. 1975; Piotrowski et al. 1975; Clark, Hench and Paschall 1976) with silica-based glass-ceramic implants has shown that the surface chemistry of the implant, particularly the phosphorus content, influences the response of the surrounding bone. A certain phosphorus content resulted in co-crystallisation between the bone and the implant, with an interface strength higher than that of the bulk implant and approaching that of the bone. Whether such phosphorus-containing glasses would be as suitable in other respects as alumina, or whether the two could be combined, remains to be seen; but the idea of effecting incorporation of an implant by control of its surface chemistry is of fundamental importance.

4 MEASUREMENTS OF STRENGTH OF FIXATION

Having considered the relevant basic information and its implications for the design of interfaces, it is appropriate to review the measurements which have been made of the strengths achieved using representative prosthetic components implanted in bone.

4.1 Hip Prostheses

4.1.1 FEMORAL COMPONENTS

Al Habooby (1969) applied compressive loads to five Charnley femoral components cemented into cadaveric femora. Bones with prostheses failed by fracture of the bone at loads within the range of failing loads measured on intact femora by Frankel (1960). Grünert and Ritter (1973) applied cyclic compressive loads to Müller femoral head prostheses cemented into fresh cadaveric bones. After 10 cycles at the lowest range of load the maximum and minimum load were both increased, 10 further cycles were applied, and so on until loosening or fracture occurred. Thus the full significance of the results is not conveyed by a simple statement of the loads at failure, but for the present purpose it may be noted that in a femur from a 62-year-old female loosening occurred during cycling to a maximum load of 5 000 N, whereas in 'strong, younger bones' cycling at loads up to 5 000 N produced no visible effects, and static loads up to about 12 000 N were needed to produce failure, which was by splitting of the bone.

For comparison, the peak load imposed on a hip joint in level walking would usually be between three and five times body weight (Paul 1967). With a body mass of 70 kg, this would correspond to about 2 100 N if walking gently (as most patients with prosthetic joints may be expected to), or about 3 500 N if walking fairly vigorously.

The femoral component of the ICLH hip prosthesis, which consists of a part-spherical metallic cap having a cylindrical bore which is cemented to the femoral neck after this has been cut to size, has been tested in the author's laboratory by Day. Five femora fitted with the prosthetic head failed by breaking of the bone (usually subcapitally, close to the distal end of the cap) at loads between 3 720 and 8 530 N, the average being 6 670 N. Two intact femora failed at 9 400 and 9 500 N respectively; these were paired with two of those tested after prosthetic replacement, which failed at 6 670 and 8 530 N respectively. Thus it appears that the strength of the femoral neck is reduced by approximately 10–30 per cent by the interruption of the cortex involved in this operation. The lowest strength measured, 3 720 N, is less than twice the peak load (2 100 N) mentioned above as corresponding to a body mass of 70 kg in gentle walking, and this margin might be unsafe when considering the possibility of fatigue fracture (the femur in question was from an 87-year-old female with a body mass of 45 kg, which may well have been lower than the body mass before the terminal illness).

The results of these few tests suggest firstly that the fixation of both stemmed and stemless femoral components is stronger than the bone, that the strength of the bone is reduced from that of an intact femoral head and neck by the necessary cutting, and that the strength of the bone-prosthesis system will usually be at least three times the peak force likely to be exerted in level walking by most patients fitted with total hip replacement prostheses.

The fixation of acetabular components has been tested by Andersson, Freeman and Swanson (1972), Chen et al. (1974), Halleux, Duriau and Blaimont (1974), and Jäger et al. (1974). Andersson, Freeman and Swanson and Chen et al. used one or more standard designs of acetabular cup implanted into fresh cadaveric specimens, and found that the torsional strength of the cement–bone interface was greater than the frictional moment measured in any hip prosthesis, although Andersson, Freeman and Swanson pointed out that the margin of strength was sometimes low enough to make fatigue failure of the bone a possibility in clinical practice (failure occurred on the bone side of the bone–cement interface). Jäger et al. used a special cup with unusually large external fins, to ensure that failure occurred at the cement–bone interface, and obtained results similar to those of the other authors. Halleux's group used a simulated acetabular cup, and measured the torsional strengths of the cement–bone interface after different methods of preparing the acetabular surface. They found that acetabula prepared by simply removing the cartilage were weaker than those in which holes were made and filled with cement, and regarded this difference in strength as important. Jäger et al. also attach importance to the increased strength obtained by drilling holes about 9 mm in diameter and 20 mm deep into the pubis, ilium and ischium, whereas Chen et al. and Andersson, Freeman and Swanson considered this increase unnecessary and perhaps not worth the possible penalty resulting from increased interference with the mechanical integrity and blood supply of the bone; these two groups considered the strength obtained by decortication and thorough roughening of the cancellous bone to be sufficient. This view may be compared with the clinical observations of Münzenberg and Dennert (1975), who report that since they stopped opening the cancellous space of the acetabular bone in patients with advanced osteoporosis they have not seen aseptic loosening.

Against all these measurements can be made the two criticisms that the torsional moments were applied about the axis of symmetry of the cup, which is not the axis about which the greatest frictional moments are likely to be applied in life, and that they reflect the strength of the interface at the time of implantation and not as it may be modified by changes occurring afer implantation (although Andersson, Freeman and Swanson did test also one specimen which had been implanted for two years). The latter criticism is more important in view of the observations, discussed above and in Chapter 4, of fibrous membranes established between bone and cement one or more years after implantation. If, as seems possible, irregularities of about 1 mm in depth are taken up by this membrane instead of being filled with bone, the consequences for a part-spherical interface without major projections would be serious. Further work is needed here, and may show the need for substantial departures from a regular hemispherical surface for the bone–cement interface.

4.2 Knee Prostheses

Nogi et al. (1976) tested three Polycentric and three Geomedic (or Geometric) knee prostheses implanted into knees obtained at amputation for vascular disease. Compressive loads were applied along the axis of the femoral shaft, with the tibia held rigidly in either full extension or 20° flexion. Some specimens failed under compressive load, some under compressive load combined with rotation of the femur about its long axis (which transferred the load to one or other condyle), and some under repeatedly applied compressive load. The three Polycentric prostheses failed by crushing of the cancellous bone under the tibial component, at compressive loads of 637–2 720 N. The three Geomedic prostheses failed by disruption of the bone–cement interface under the tibial component at loads of between 1 827 and 3 230 N. The application of rotation, without measuring the consequent redistribution of forces, combined with the fact that different tests were performed successively on the same specimens, makes these results a little difficult to interpret, but the failing loads can be compared with peak forces of three times body weight (Morrison 1970); i.e. about 2 100 N for a body mass of 70 kg.

Experiments by Day, Yamamoto and Bargren in the author's laboratory have measured the strengths of four designs of knee prostheses (the Geomedic, ICLH, Marmor, and Total Condylar) in compression, torsion and hyperextension, and have compared these strengths with the loads that can be transmitted through the natural knee in healthy subjects. With compressive loads applied centrally to the tibial components through the femoral components or similarly shaped pads, crushing of the cancellous bone occurred at loads between 3 000 and 15 400 N. The results showed the importance of engaging the tibial cortex as well as the cancellous bone. Compression applied eccentrically in a lateral or medial sense gave failure at significantly lower loads. In torsion, the results showed clearly how the resistance of a prosthetic knee depends on the geometry of the articulating surfaces; designs in which a concave tibial surface caused the femoral component to rise as it was rotated induced more tension in the collateral ligaments and were therefore stiffer in torsion than the one design tested (Marmor) which had a more nearly flat tibial surface. All the specimens tested dislocated without damaging the fixation when torsion was combined with a vertical compressive load equal to body weight. In hyperextension, all four designs of prosthesis failed at bending moments between one-half and two-thirds as high as the average measured on four natural knees. The failing moment of the prosthetic knees (51–67 Nm) may be compared with hyperextending moments of 40 Nm supported by muscular effort by young adults.

4.3 Ankle Prostheses

Kempson, Freeman and Tuke (1975) published the results of torsional tests on the ICLH ankle prosthesis. Under a constant vertical compressive force of 1 800 N, four natural ankles failed (by avulsion of a ligament from a malleolus) at twisting moments between 40 and 63 Nm; four ankles in which the prosthesis had been implanted failed, also by avulsion of a ligament from a malleolus, at moments between 29 and 40 Nm. Three of each group were paired; i.e. from the same cadaver. Little is known of the twisting moments applied to ankles in life, but these results were compared with moments of about 22 Nm which caused pain in healthy young adults. The authors inferred that failure in torsion is unlikely to occur in life.

4.4 Summary

These test results on prostheses for three different joints show that the fixation can, in some circumstances, be made to be stronger than the bone, and that the loads needed to cause failure, whilst in general lower than for the corresponding natural joint, are higher than either the loads arising at the relevant joints in normal walking (where these are known) or the loads which can be exerted by muscular action in young adults. The margin of static strength over the probable service loads may not always be large enough to ensure freedom from fatigue failure in the bone, and this emphasises the importance of keeping the stresses in the bone as low as possible by engaging the whole of the available cross-section, including the cortex.

5 METHYL METHACRYLATE AS A BONDING AGENT

5.1 Limitations of Methyl Methacrylate

It is well known that polymethylmethacrylate has disadvantages as a bonding agent: the methyl methacrylate monomer is toxic; the necessary additives may be toxic; the insertion of a plug as firmly as possible into the medullary cavity tends to force fat into the circulatory system; hypotension and cardiac arrest have occasionally been experienced a few minutes after inserting acrylic cement; the polymerisation of methyl methacrylate is exothermic and accompanied by a volumetric shrinkage of about 4 per cent (Ohnsorge and Grötz, 1974); its stiffness differs from that of bone; and the removal of cement, particularly from a long intramedullary site, may be extremely difficult. A further possible disadvantage which has more recently become apparent and which is discussed in Chapter 4, is that a degree of loosening which in itself might be tolerable can permit abrasion of cement against bone with the production of particulate debris, and that this debris may cause bone necrosis thereby making the loosening progressive.

Some of these disadvantages are theoretical and others are matters of observation in practice. Some are peculiar to methyl methacrylate whilst others might be common to some or all other cements. Whilst all of them must be seen against the background of a high rate of clinical success, the desire to eliminate failures has led to investigations of each of these undesirable features of methyl methacrylate cement, and to the search for other cements.

Biological reactions to acrylic cement, including the effects of the temperatures likely to be reached during polymerisation, are discussed in Chapter 4. The following discussion is concerned with the mechanical aspects of the factors listed above.

5.2 Stiffness

Young's modulus in compression of methacrylate polymerised in industrial conditions is about 3 GN/m^2; for the cement polymerised *in situ* the effective value is likely to be lower, depending on the degree of aeration, inclusion of foreign matter, etc. Buchholz and Engelbrecht (1970) obtained values of $1 \cdot 6 - 1 \cdot 7 \text{ GN/m}^2$ from bending tests on bone cement mixed as it would be clinically but not exposed to tissues. These values are compared in Table 5.2 with typical values for compact and cancellous bone, and for materials used in prostheses. The values for metallic materials are accurate to within a few per cent, but those for plastics and bone (particularly cancellous bone) are far more variable and should not be taken as better than orders of magnitude in the present context. Within these limitations, acrylic cement as normally used has a stiffness lower than both that of implantable alloys and that of compact bone, but higher

Table 5.2 Young's Moduli of Methyl Methacrylate, Bone, and Prosthesis Materials

Material	Source	Young's modulus (GN/m²)
Methyl methacrylate, polymerised in industrial conditions	Manufacturers' literature	c.3
Methyl methacrylate mixed and polymerised in clinical conditions (but not contaminated)	Buchholz and Engelbrecht (1970)	1·6–1·7
Compact bone	Swanson (1971)	10–20
Cancellous bone	Yokoo (1952)	0·09
Austenitic stainless steel		190
Co–Cr–Mo alloy		200
Titanium		100
Polyethylene (not high molecular weight)	Manufacturers' literature	0·7

than that of cancellous bone and slightly higher than that of polyethylene.

An optimum value would be between that of the implant and that of the bone, but closer to the latter because relative movement between implant and cement is less harmful than between cement and bone. Clearly, no one cement can achieve this for all the possible combinations (metal in tubular compact bone, metal in cancellous bone, plastic in tubular compact bone, plastic in cancellous bone). The effective stiffness of cement can be reduced by aerating it during mixing, and this and other methods are being examined for possible clinical use; but, if it were thought to be desirable to achieve more than a rough approximation, such methods would make clinical practice appreciably more complicated. Cements other than methyl methacrylate, some of which may offer a different stiffness, are considered below.

5.3 Addition of Antibiotics

The prevention and treatment of infection are outside the scope of this chapter, but notice must be taken of the method of treatment and prophylaxis based on the addition of antibiotics to the cement, suggested and used clinically by Buchholz and Engelbrecht (1970). Hessert and Ruckdeschel (1970) found that, of various antibiotic powders, gentamicin was released in significant quantities *in vitro* in 24 hours and had a usefully broad spectrum of activity. Hessert (1971) showed that the tensile strength of Palacos acrylic cement was not significantly reduced by the addition of up to 2 g of gentamicin sulphate to the standard pack of 40 g of powder and 20 g of liquid. The matter was discussed by Koschmieder, Ritzerfeld and Kleymann (1973), Schulitz and Schöning (1973), Wizgall (1973) and by Levin (1975), all of whom were concerned with the bactericidal effects and not with the possible mechanical disadvantages. The latter seem, on the basis of Hessert's results, to be unlikely to be important.

6 CEMENTS OTHER THAN METHYL METHACRYLATE

Cements other than methyl methacrylate have been considered. These have included butyl methacrylate either as a polymer or as a copolymer with methyl methacrylate, cyclohexyl methacrylate as a copolymer with methyl methacrylate (de Wijn 1974), zinc poly-carboxylate (Friend 1969; Peters et al. 1972; Peters, Jackson and Smith 1974), and silicone elastomer (Kenesi and Lortat-Jacob 1973). The last-named has been used in plastic and maxillofacial surgery for some time, and its compatibility with body tissues in those conditions of use is therefore known. Zinc polycarboxylate (known also as zinc polyacrylic) cement has been used for some time in dentistry, and therefore is also known to be biocompatible in some circumstances; but those circumstances have not been such as to require any knowledge of the heat evolved in its polymerisation or of its mechanical properties when polymerised in masses of tens of grams, several millimetres thick. The same is true of other dental cements already or potentially in use, such as glass ionomers (Kent, Lewis and Wilson 1973).

A less radical departure from present practice is that of using methyl methacrylate with a different catalyst, tri-n-butylborane, which, according to Iida et al. (1974), gives a lower polymerisation temperature and improved strength, the latter resulting from a chemical bond to bone collagen. These authors reported clinical use at the hip with follow-up to about two years, and histological observations in rats up to one year after implantation of non-load-bearing plugs of cement in the femoral medullary cavity. New bone formation around the cement was seen, but it is not clear whether the bonding to collagen, achieved during polymerisation, was preserved.

It is instructive to look at the search for other cements in the light of the known limitations to the long-term performance of methyl methacrylate.

The stiffness of methyl methacrylate is already of orders of magnitude lower than those of metallic materials, of the same order of magnitude as that of polyethylene, and between those of compact and cancellous bone. In view of this, and of the wide variations in properties of cement exposed to contamination with blood and air, there seems no point in seeking a cement with a different stiffness.

The remodelling of bone and the formation of a fibrous layer next to methyl methacrylate may be caused partly by the temperature reached during polymerisation or by a reaction to the monomer, and to this extent a change of cement might be useful. However, a similar fibrous layer was observed by Biehl, Harms and Mäusle (1975) adjacent to a serrated metal stem implanted without cement, and this makes it seem unlikely that the reaction is specific to methyl methacrylate. This topic is discussed more fully in Chapter 4, section 2.2.

The possibility that abraded particles of methyl methacrylate cause bone necrosis and consequent progressive loosening, if it were proven, would invite further investigations to discover whether particles of other cements produced the same effects; for it must be accepted that with any cement on some occasions slight loosening will occur which is not itself of clinical significance but which will allow particles of bone or cement or both to be abraded.

7 SUMMARY

Absolute rigidity of fixation is unattainable; the looseness to be avoided is that which progressively increases to a level giving pain or disability.

Histology shows that about two years after implantation the bone adjacent to an implant undergoes fibrous replacement, the fibrous tissue having a thickness varying up to 1·5 mm and tending to fill any asperities in the implant surface. A fibrous membrane has been observed around both cemented and uncemented implants.

Assuming this layer of fibrous tissue to be weak in tension and shear but able to transmit compression, it follows that prostheses should be designed so that significant tensile and shear stresses do not arise at the interfaces with bone, whether cement be used or not.

Natural joints transmit mainly compression through their articular surfaces, and tension and torsion through their ligaments. A prosthetic joint which replaces the functions of the ligaments as well as those of the articular surfaces will therefore transmit tensile and torsion loads to its interfaces with bone. Since such loads are likely to produce tensile and shear stresses at the bone–implant interfaces, prostheses should as far as possible replace joint surfaces, not ligaments. Tensile and torsion loads on the interface can be limited by so shaping the articulating surfaces that above a certain load spontaneously reducing subluxations are permitted in ordinary use. Overloads would then be expected to cause subluxation rather than loosening.

Given that however the articulating surfaces are designed some tensile and torsion loads will be transmitted across the bone–prosthesis interfaces, these loads can be transmitted mainly by means of compressive stresses if mechanical interlocking is provided. To minimise these compressive stresses and also those corresponding to compressive loads, the largest practicable area of interface should be provided. This can be done by shaping the relevant surfaces of the prosthetic components appropriately.

It is not usually practicable to arrange for interlocking shapes on the prosthetic components to be engaged with strong bone at the time of implantation, and some temporary fixation is needed if the shapes alone, without cement, are relied on.

Cement allows interlocking to be achieved at the time of implantation and increases the area of contact (thus decreasing the stresses on the interface) by filling gaps between the bone and the prosthesis. In view of the remodelling of bone adjacent to surface features up to about 1 mm deep, interlock should be provided by features in the bone surface several millimetres deep, either filled with cement or occupied by corresponding features on the prosthesis surface surrounded by a thin layer of cement.

Bone ingrowth into rough or porous surfaces offers another way of achieving interlock in conjunction with suitable gross shapes of the surfaces, but to achieve bone ingrowth it seems likely that the prosthesis must be immobilised in the bone for the few months needed for bone to grow into the holes. This may be difficult to achieve if the patient is allowed to bear weight on an uncemented prosthesis; and it is not yet known whether bone which has grown in while the prosthesis is unloaded will be replaced by fibrous tissue when weight-bearing is resumed.

Methyl methacrylate cement as now used is not an ideal material but in practice its defects are not serious, and which of them are specific to this cement and which would be shared by other cements, is not certain.

REFERENCES

Al Habooby, S. (1969) Load transfer from prosthesis to bone. *M.Sc. Dissertation*, University of Manchester, Institute of Science and Technology.

Amstutz, H. C., Lurie, L. and Bullough, P. (1972) Skeletal fixation with self-curing polymethylmethacrylate. A report of 23 canine total hip replacements. *Clinical Orthopaedics and Related Research* **84**, 163.

Andersson, G. B. J., Freeman, M. A. R. and Swanson S. A. V. (1972) Loosening of the cemented acetabular cup in total hip replacement. *Journal of Bone and Joint Surgery* **54B**, 590.

Biehl, G., Harms, J. and Mäusle E. (1975) Tierexperimentelle und histopathologische Untersuchungen über die Anpassungsvorgänge des Knochens nach der Implantation von 'Tragrippen-Endoprothesen'. *Archiv für Orthopädische und Unfall-Chirurgie* **81**, 105.

Boutin, P. (1972) Arthroplastie total de la hanche par prothèse en alumine frittée. *Revue de Chirurgie Orthopédique et Reparatrice de l'Appareil Moteur* **58**, 229.

Boutin, P. (1974) Les prothèses totales de la hanche en alumine. L'ancrage direct sans ciment dans 50 cas. *Revue de Chirurgie Orthopédique et Reparatrice de l'Appareil Moteur* **60**, 233.

Buchholz, H. W. and Engelbrecht, H. (1970) Über die Depotwirkung einiger Antibiotica bei Vermischung mit dem Kunstharz Palacos. *Der Chirurg* **41**, 511.

Cameron, H. U., Pilliar, R. M. and MacNab, I. (1973) The effect of movement on the bonding of porous metal to bone. *Journal of Biomedical Materials Research* **7**, 301.

Charnley, J. (1970) *Acrylic Cement in Orthopaedic Surgery*. Edinburgh and London, Churchill Livingstone.

Chen, S. C., Lowe, S. A., Scales, J. T. and Ansell, R. H. (1974) An in vitro experiment to determine the efficiency of fixation of the McKee–Farrar acetabular component in relation to torsional force. *Acta Orthopaedica Scandinavica* **45**, 429.

Clark, A. E., Hench, L. L. and Paschall, H. A. (1976) The influence of surface chemistry on implant interface histology: A theoretical basis for implant materials selection. *Journal of Biomedical Materials Research* **10**, 161.

Frankel, V. H. (1960) *The Femoral Neck: an experimental study of function, fracture mechanism and internal fixation*. Stockholm, Almquist and Wiksell.

Friend, L. A. (1969) Handling properties of a zinc polycarboxylate cement. An investigation. *British Dental Journal* **127**, 359.

Galante, J., Rostoker, W., Lueck, R. and Ray, D. (1971) Sintered fiber metal composites as a basis for attachment of implants to bone. *Journal of Bone and Joint Surgery* **53A**, 101.

Griss, P., Heimke, G. and Andrian-Werburg, H. Frhr v. (1975) Die Aluminiumoxidkeramik-Metall-Verbundprothese. Eine neue Hüftgelenktotalendoprothese zur teilweise zementfreien Implantation. *Archiv für Orthopädische und Unfall-Chirurgie* **81**, 259.

Grünert, A. and Ritter, G. (1973) Experimentelle Untersuchungen zum

Problem der Verankerung von Hüftendoprothesen. *Archiv für Ortho-pädische und Unfall-Chirurgie* **77,** 149.

Halleux, P., Duriau, F. and Blaimont, P. (1974) Etude comparée de dif-férents modes d'ancrage cotyloïdien dans l'arthroplastie de la hanche. *Acta Orthopaedica Belgica* **40,** 712.

Hench, L. L., Paschall, H. A., Allen, W. C. and Piotrowski, G. (1975) National Bureau of Standards Special Publication 415, p. 19.

Hessert, G. R. (1971) Bruchfestigkeit und Struktur des Knochenzementes Palacos nach Zusatz von Gentamycin-Sulfat. *Archiv für Orthopädische und Unfall-Chirurgie* **69,** 289.

Hessert, G. R. and Ruckdeschel, G. (1970) Antibiotische Wirksamkeit von Mischungen des Polymethylmethacrylates mit Antibiotica. *Archiv für Orthopädische und Unfall-Chirurgie* **68,** 249.

Hulbert, S. F., Matthews, J. R., Klawitter, J. J., Sauer, B. W. and Leonard, R. B. (1974) Effect of stress on tissue ingrowth into porous aluminium oxide. *Journal of Biomedical Materials Research, Symposium No. 5,* part 1, p. 85.

Iida, M., Furuya, K., Kawachi, S., Masuhara, A. and Tarumi, J. (1974) New improved bone cement (MMA-TBB). *Clinical Orthopaedics and Related Research* **100,** 279.

Jäger, M., Küsswetter, W., Rütt, J. and Ungethüm, M. (1974) Experimen-telle Torsionslockerung technisch verschieden implantierter Hüftendo-prothesenpfannen. *Zeitschrift für Orthopädie und ihre Grenzgebiete* **112,** 34.

Kempson, G. E., Freeman, M. A. R. and Tuke, M. A. (1975) Engineering considerations in the design of an ankle joint. *Biomedical Engineering* **10,** 166.

Kenesi, C. and Lortat-Jacob, A. (1973) Le scellement aux silicones des prosthèses de Moore. *Revue de Chirurgie Orthopédique et Reparatrice de l'Appareil Moteur* **59,** 469.

Kent, B. E., Lewis, B. G. and Wilson, A. D. (1973) The properties of a glass ionomer cement. *British Dental Journal* **135,** 322.

Koschmieder, R., Ritzerfeld, W. and Kleymann, H. (1973) Infektionspro-phylaxe beim alloplastichen Gelenkersatz durch Gentamycinzusatz zum Polymethylmethacrylat. Tierexperimentelle Untersuchungen. *Zeitschrift für Orthopädie und ihre Grenzgebiete* **111,** 244.

Lembert, E., Galante, J. and Rostoker, W. (1972) Fixation of skeletal replacement by fiber metal composites. *Clinical Orthopaedics and Related Research* **87,** 303.

Levin, P. D. (1975) The effectiveness of various antibiotics in the methyl-methacrylate. *Journal of Bone and Joint Surgery* **57B,** 234.

Lyng, S., Sudmann, E., Hulbert, S. F. and Sauer, B. W. (1973) Fixation of permanent orthopaedic prostheses. Use of ceramics in the tibial plateau. *Acta Orthopaedica Scandinavica* **44,** 694.

Mittelmeier, H. (1974) Zementlose Verankerung von Endoprothesen nach dem Tragrippenprinzip. *Zeitschrift für Orthopädie und ihre Grenzge-biete* **112,** 27.

Morrison, J. B. (1970) Biomechanics of the knee joint in relation to normal walking. *Journal of Biomechanics* **3,** 51.

Münzenberg, K. J. and Dennert, R. (1975) Pfannenlockerung bei Hüfttotal-endoprothesen infolge altersabhängigen Knochensubstanzverlustes. *Zeit-schrift für Orthopädie und ihre Grenzgebiete* **113,** 947.

Nilles, J. L., Coletti, J. M. Jr. and Wilson, C. (1973) Biomechanical evalu-ation of bone–porous material interfaces. *Journal of Biomedical Materials Research* **7,** 231.

Nogi, J., Caldwell, J. W., Kauzlarich, J. J. and Thomson, R. C. (1976) Load testing of Geometric and Polycentric total knee replacements. *Clinical Orthopaedics and Related Research* **114,** 235.

Ohnsorge, J. and Grötz, J. (1974) Dimensionsänderung des aushärtenden

Knochenzementes. *Zeitschrift für Orthopädie und ihre Grenzgebiete* **112**, 975.

Paul, J. P. (1967) Forces transmitted by joints in the human body. *Proceedings, Institution of Mechanical Engineers* **181** (3J), 8.

Peters, W. J., Jackson, R. W. and Smith, D. C. (1974) Studies of the stability and toxicity of zinc polyacrylate (polycarboxylate) cements (PAZ). *Journal of Biomedical Materials Research* **8**, 53.

Peters, W. J., Jackson, R. W., Iwano, K. and Smith, D. C. (1972) The biological response to zinc polyacrylate cement. *Clinical Orthopaedics and Related Research* **88**, 228.

Piotrowski, G., Hench, L. L., Allen, W. C. and Miller, G. J. (1975) Mechanical studies of the bone bioglass interfacial bond. *Journal of Biomedical Materials Research, Symposium No. 6*, p. 47.

Ring, P. A. (1968) Complete replacement arthroplasty of the hip by the Ring prosthesis. *Journal of Bone and Joint Surgery* **50B**, 720.

Schulitz, K. P. and Schöning, B. (1973) Antibioticazusatz zum Knochenzement oder nicht? *Archiv für Orthopädische und Unfall-Chirurgie* **77**, 31.

Sivash, K. M. (1969) The development of a total metal prosthesis for the hip joint from a partial joint replacement. *Reconstruction Surgery and Traumatology* **11**, 53.

Swanson, S. A. V. (1971) Biomechanical characteristics of bone. In, *Advances in Biomedical Engineering*, Vol. 1, p. 137. Ed. R. M. Kenedi. New York and London, Academic Press.

Welsh, R. P., Pilliar, R. M. and MacNab, I. (1971) Surgical implants: the role of surface porosity in fixation to bone and acrylic. *Journal of Bone and Joint Surgery* **53A**, 963.

de Wijn, J. R. (1974) Reduction of maximum temperature in the polymerization of cold- and heat-curing acrylic resins. *Journal of Biomedical Materials Research* **8**, 421.

Willert, H.-G. and Puls, P. (1972) Die Reaktion des Knochens auf Knochenzement bei der Allo-Arthroplastik der Hüft. *Archiv für Orthopädische und Unfall-Chirurgie* **72**, 33.

Willert, H.-G., Ludwig, J. and Semlitsch, M. (1974) Reaction of bone to methacrylate after hip arthroplasty. A long-term gross, light microscopic and scanning electron microscopic study. *Journal of Bone and Joint Surgery* **56A**, 1368.

Wizgall, J. (1973) Vergleichende Untersuchungen bei der Implantation von Hüftgelenkstotalprothesen. *Archiv für Orthopädische und Unfall-Chirurgie* **75**, 65.

Yokoo, S. (1952) Compression test of the cancellated bone. *Journal of Kyoto Prefectural Medical University* **51**, 273.

CHAPTER SIX

Manufacture

1 PURPOSE OF THIS CHAPTER

THIS chapter does not set out to describe completely the manufacture of prostheses, which would be neither practicable nor necessary. It would not be practicable because, although the main processes are generally known, the details of their application are known in the form of accumulations of experience in a limited number of manufacturers' establishments, this being one field of manufacture in which success requires attention to a large amount of detailed technique as well as a knowledge of the principles involved. It is not necessary because most readers of this book will be users and not makers of joint replacement prostheses. Many readers will, of course, be potential or actual designers of prostheses, and the main purpose of this chapter is to describe the manufacturing process in sufficient detail to enable designers and users to appreciate the ways in which the processes of manufacture are related to those of design.

2 METALLIC COMPONENTS

2.1 General Outline

For all metallic components, the sequence of operations is the same, consisting of the following processes:

> production of the alloy in bulk;
> shaping of the component;
> accurate forming where required;
> finishing of surfaces;
> marking;
> packing.

Some of these processes are the same, or nearly so, for all the alloys now used, but others take different forms with different alloys. The chief differences are in the means employed to shape the component from the alloy in bulk. Two considerations govern the choice of means of shaping the implant. Economically, to machine large numbers of components from the solid alloy would be expensive in time and in waste metal, and it is cheaper to go to the initial trouble of setting up equipment to produce the approximate shape either by deforming the metal while hot (forging) or melting it and recasting it into the desired shape. Functionally, the crystal size and structure in a cast billet do not usually give the best mechanical properties in the final component, having regard to the directions in which it may be stressed. The crystal structure can be modified by plastically deforming the metal; cold deformation is suitable for some purposes, but is not practicable for the present purpose; and hot plastic deformation (forging) is used for stainless steel and titanium alloys. The cobalt–chromium alloy used for bearing surfaces ('cast cobalt–chromium', Table 1.1, known commercially by such names as Vitallium, Vinertia, Alivium, Protasul 2) is too brittle at all usable temperatures to make forging practicable, and is therefore remelted and cast into the shapes of individual components.

2.2 Production of the Alloy in Bulk

Essentially, this process consists of mixing the required constituents in the molten state and, of course, the exclusion of unwanted constituents ('impurities'). The limits on the permitted quantities of some constituents are tight, sometimes less than one-tenth of 1 per cent of the total mass, so the process is by no means simple. It is also important that the constituents should be uniformly distributed, within close limits, throughout the bulk (one consequence of failure to achieve this is the corrosion which sometimes occurs when neighbouring regions of the surface react differently in the presence of saline solutions). Homogeneity of constituents must, of course, be preserved through the later processes, which usually involve the production of several components from one billet of alloy.

These standards of accuracy and purity are attained by processes more complicated than those which suffice for making mild steel for motor cars or animal feeding troughs, or cast iron for drain-pipes. More than one melting, perhaps in a vacuum furnace, is usual, and the general standard of cleanliness needs to be higher than usually associated with foundries. Thus the alloys used for surgical implants, like those for critical applications in other branches of engineering, are produced in a small number of plants, typically one or two per alloy (because producers tend to specialise in titanium or alloy steels or cobalt alloys) in any one technologically advanced country.

2.3 Forging of Steel and Titanium Alloys

Stainless steel and titanium alloys are made into the required shape by hot forging, i.e. by pressing the material between shaped dies at a temperature which makes the alloy easier to deform than when cold and, more importantly, ensures that crystals are able to re-form in ways imposed by the forming process. The flow of metal from its original shape into that of the inside of the dies, correctly co-ordinated with the control of temperature, produces a crystal structure which gives the best combination of properties. A badly designed or badly executed forging process can give properties other than those intended: perhaps an excessive brittleness, excessive directional variation of mechanical properties, or local segregation of alloying constituents. Some shapes can be made in one operation; others require two or more stages, with dies of intermediate shape, and reheating for each stage.

Forging can produce shapes with dimensional accuracy of about ±0·25 mm, which means that parts whose dimensions are not critical need a surface smoothing treatment but not a precision finishing process. Bearing surfaces need machining or grinding to achieve the necessary accuracy.

As the component leaves the forging dies, the crystal structure will vary between different parts, because different parts will have deformed to different extents. Particularly with stainless steel, such regional variations can increase the susceptibility to corrosion in the body (see Chapter 1, section 1.5), and it is therefore usual to anneal forgings; i.e. to heat them to a temperature at which crystals re-form to an extent sufficient to remove the effects of plastic deformation. The penalty of this is that the yield and ultimate strengths of the material are reduced, and since even a few fatigue fractures in service (see Chapter 1, section 2.3) show that in some circumstances there is no margin of strength, the best way to treat forgings at this stage of their manufacture is still being discussed.

2.4 Investment Casting of Cobalt–Chromium Alloys

A mould is made, having a cavity of the shape of the component, with allowances for shrinkage during cooling and for metal to be removed by grinding where this is needed for dimensional accuracy.

This mould is used to make wax models of the component. As many wax models are needed as components; thus if 1 000 components of one design are to be made, rather more than 1 000 wax models will be made, to allow for wastage and samples for destruction testing.

About 20 wax models are assembled, connected by branches to a common trunk. This assembly is then sprayed with several coats of a paste containing a refractory powder. The first coat contains very fine powder, so that every detail of the assembly is closely invested by the paste (hence the usual name of the process). Later coats are coarser, and are added in sufficient number to make the accumulation of paste, when baked, strong enough to withstand handling.

The invested wax model assemblies are then baked. During this process the refractory paste fuses to form a mould, and the wax melts and is poured out of the mould (hence another name for the process: 'lost wax'). This leaves an empty mould, containing about 20 cavities each the shape of the component, all connected to the trunk into which molten metal can be poured. Provision is also made, when assembling the wax models, for air to escape as molten metal enters. The number of wax models assembled on to one trunk depends on the size of the component and on the standard quantity of alloy melted in the casting furnace, which is generally several kilograms.

Next, molten alloy is poured into the mould which has been previously heated to a suitable temperature to prevent excessive chilling of the molten alloy as it enters the mould. When the mould has been filled, it is allowed to cool at a controlled rate.

When cool enough to ensure that the alloy has solidified, the mould is broken away mechanically, leaving a number of components all joined to the common trunk. The components are then broken or cut off, and the surplus alloy removed from the places where metal ran into each component-shaped cavity.

This process may seem wasteful in labour and material, but it can produce components with a dimensional accuracy of ± 0.05 mm. For many purposes, no further removal of metal is then needed, which is a particular advantage with an alloy which is difficult to machine. One mould (usually made in metal and expensive) can produce thousands of wax models, and the making of these is a low-energy process compared with that of forging steel or titanium alloys. Careful control is needed all through the process, but the equipment, other than that for making the wax models, is relatively simple, and consumable materials (wax and refractory paste) are relatively cheap.

Cobalt–chromium alloy components are generally heat-treated after casting and trimming, to reduce the brittleness of the material.

2.5 Accurate Forming of Component

Whether the component has been forged or cast, bearing surfaces must be accurately shaped before being polished, and other surfaces may also need further shaping if, for example, intramedullary stems are to have cross-sectional dimensions controlled to tight tolerances to ensure interchangeability in the patient. None of the alloys in question is easy to machine; cutting tools tend to tear material off stainless steel and titanium alloys instead of separating it cleanly, while cobalt–chromium alloys are too hard to be machined using alloy steel tools and require ceramic cutting edges on the tools. Unless considerable amounts of metal are to be removed, grinding is often preferred to machining for cobalt–chromium alloys.

Special-purpose machine tools are used as necessary (e.g. those which generate spherical surfaces) and some automation is common when long runs of one component are required.

2.6 Finishing of Surfaces

For the finishing of non-bearing surfaces, practices vary, and the variation seems to result partly from functional and partly from aesthetic considerations. Function requires that all surfaces be smooth enough to eliminate all crevices or blemishes which could act as stress concentrations or foci of corrosion. Beyond this is an element of choice. A mirror finish looks attractive, a satin finish is as attractive, and a roughened or textured finish is likely to offer a better key for cement than either.

The necessary smoothing is usually achieved with abrasive paper or cloth, either as a moving belt against which flat or convex parts of the component are held or, for concave parts, as small hand-held rotating cylinders driven by flexible shafts. Polishing is by abrasion, using successively finer abrasives, or by electrolytic means. Rough surfaces can be produced by sand blasting, and textured surfaces by applying a textured surface to the wax model if investment casting is used, or (less easily) to the forging dies.

Titanium and stainless steel components are finally treated in nitric acid, partly in order to ensure the presence of a strong oxide film for corrosion resistance (see Chapter 1, section 1.5), and partly in order to remove any ferrous particles which may remain from earlier processes.

Bearing surfaces are finished by abrasion, using successively finer abrasives until the surface roughness is reduced to typically 0·025–0·05 μm. Traditionally, this was done by hand, the component being held against rotating calico mops charged with abrasive pastes. Excellent surface finish can be obtained by skilled operators in this way, but an unusual degree of skill is required if the dimensional tolerances are to be held to the tight ranges usually prescribed for bearing surfaces. It has therefore been necessary to develop special machines which will finish bearing surfaces to the combination of dimensional accuracy (commonly $\pm 12\cdot5$ μm) and surface roughness generally specified. The development of such a machine is reasonably straightforward if part-spherical surfaces are required, as on hip prostheses, but much less straightforward, tending to impossible, if irregular shapes such as imitations of natural condyles in knees are needed.

2.7 Marking of Components

Components must be marked to show the maker's name, the material and any information, such as the size of a femoral head, needed by the surgeon, and should carry a serial number, though this is not yet a universal practice. The marking can be done in ways that damage the component or jeopardise its long-term safety, as by indenting letters into it in a region of tensile stress in service; thus some control should be exercised over the site and method of marking.

2.8 Packing

Obviously, components must be packed so that they are not damaged in transport or storage. Since metallic components are sterilised by heat at the time of use, packing arrangements which preserve sterility are not required.

2.9 Implications for Designers and Users

Both forging and casting impose certain restrictions on the shapes of components, particularly of components likely to be highly stressed in a corrosive environment. Sharp corners, which are undesirable because they act as stress concentrations and may increase the chances of fatigue failure (see Chapter 1, section 1.4), would anyway be difficult to make by either forging or casting. Large variations in thickness of material cause difficulties in either forging or casting (because of the different rates of cooling and therefore of shrinkage), and are best avoided. Thus in hip prostheses cast in cobalt–chromium alloy, the larger sizes of ball are made hollow to avoid the large mass of a solid ball; this requires that they be made in two parts and welded (which process is allowed in these alloys but not in stainless steel because in this alloy it tends to produce non-uniform distribution of the chromium content and hence a greater susceptibility to corrosive attack). Forging dies and the moulds for making wax models have to be made in two or more parts which are separated to release the component or model, and this separation is made more difficult if the shape includes surfaces exactly parallel to the direction of separation; nominally parallel surfaces should preferably taper by a few degrees to facilitate smooth separation and release. Re-entrant shapes can be made only within severe limits, unless a mould or die is made with three or more parts which are withdrawn in different directions. This technique is used in other industries for the moulding of plastics and the die-casting of aluminium alloys but the expense makes it less suitable for an industry producing relatively small numbers of many different designs.

For each component, a set of forging dies or a mould is required, and in general every additional size or versions needs a different die or mould; thus a prosthesis made in four sizes, left and right, needs eight dies or moulds. When the design is settled and large numbers are needed, this may be tolerable, but while the design is being developed and modified every change may involve a new die or mould, which takes time and money (these items are made by highly skilled personnel on expensive equipment, usually in firms specialising in this work and not part of the prosthesis manufacturer's organisation). Similarly, if machining or grinding fixtures have been made for the component in question, a change in the design may require new fixtures.

It is not being suggested that the convenience of manufacturers should inhibit desirable changes; but it is suggested that designers and developers should keep a sense of proportion and make changes, as far as possible, in a planned way and in full consultation with the manufacturer.

3 PLASTIC COMPONENTS

3.1 The Nature of Plastics

Plastics are basically organic polymers, i.e. substances formed by the joining of many carbon-containing molecules to make macromolecules. In theory, components could be made by taking enough macromolecules to give the required volume and causing them to adhere to each other, but in practice other substances are usually present.

The polymerisation process involves catalysts, and to eliminate these is almost impossible although the residues may be of the order of only tens of parts per million. For general engineering use, practical plastics often contain plasticisers, fillers and colouring matter. For the present purpose, as discussed in Chapter 1, most polymers can be dismissed as unsuitable either biologically or mechanically, and the only polymer which is widely accepted, ultra-high molecular weight polyethylene, is required with the lowest practicable level of contaminants and strict control over any deliberate addition such as a plasticiser.

Polyethylene of this kind is at present available from one manufacturer in Europe and one or two in North America. This polyethylene is chemically and mechanically the same as that used for a number of special industrial purposes where chemical inertness, good mechanical properties and good wear resistance are needed; the surgical grade differs in the control exercised over its purity. The market for ultra-high molecular weight polyethylene is small by the standards of the plastics industry, and this fact, combined with the need for strict controls over material intended for implantation, has probably deterred other manufacturers from entering this particular field.

3.2 Manufacturing Sequence

The polyethylene is produced in the form of powder. This is compression-moulded, at an elevated temperature, into rectangular blocks (800 × 400 × 55 mm). Prosthetic components are machined from these blocks.

Polyethylene is machined using equipment basically similar to that used for machining metal components; special tools are used to produce particular shapes, and cutting speeds, etc. have to be suitable for the material, but nothing elaborate or unusual is required apart from the need to avoid contamination.

The above outline applies to the manufacture of most polyethylene components as now practised. If plastics other than high molecular weight polyethylene were used, it is probable that individual parts would be moulded in their final shape because, as with metallic components, if large numbers are to be made it is advantageous to put effort into the making of one mould rather than into the removal of material from each of hundreds or thousands of items. With plastics, these processes offer the further advantage of allowing the mechanical properties, including, with suitable processing, the wear resistance, to be improved during the forming process. These techniques, commonly applied to other plastics, have not so far been routinely used on high molecular weight polyethylene because at the temperatures which are allowable (too high a temperature will damage any plastic) its viscosity is too high, and the lubricants which would be used with other plastics cannot be used in this application because of the risk of contamination. Some high molecular weight polyethylene components, particularly with shapes that are not easily produced by machining, have been finally shaped, after some machining, by a hot compression-moulding technique similar to that used initially to mould powder into blocks or bars.

Some effort is being put into developing different ways of making prosthetic components in high molecular weight polyethylene, with a view both to making the process less wasteful and to improving the wear resistance of the product; over the next few years some changes in practice seem likely.

The sterilisation of polyethylene components is difficult. The temperature necessary if heat is used causes changes in shape, chemical sterilisation has dangers, and irradiation affects the mechanical properties. The present method of choice is irradiation, the permissible dose being limited to a level which changes the mechanical properties within acceptable limits. Components must be irradiated in one of a limited number of establishments having the facilities, and polyethylene components must therefore be packed so as to preserve sterility and to indicate that sterility has been preserved.

3.3 Implications

As long as plastic components are made by being machined from the solid, the restrictions imposed on the design by the manufacturing process will differ from those in the manufacture of metallic components. Machining is better suited to relatively simple shapes because compound curvatures, thin sections, or re-entrant shapes can be difficult or expensive to produce by cutting with machine tools. On the other hand, to change a feature in a design may involve changing a fixture or substituting a different tool, which is in general less expensive and quicker than making a new casting mould or forging die. If either the acceptance of a different plastic or the development of moulding techniques for high molecular weight polyethylene results in the widespread use of moulding instead of machining, then plastic components will be subject to some of the same limitations as forged metallic components. Compound curvatures will cause less difficulty (but re-entrant shapes will still be difficult), and changes of shape will require changes to dies which are expensive in money and time.

4 CERAMIC COMPONENTS

These have not yet been used widely enough for the manufacturing process to have been standardised, but the sequence of operations, long established for the making of ceramic components for other applications, must be basically the same for prosthetic components in ceramics. This sequence contains three essential steps: (1) the powder (e.g. aluminium oxide) is pressed into the shape of the component; (2) the component is heated to the temperature (c. 1 600–1 800°C) needed to fuse the powder into one continuous mass; and (3) any bearing surfaces are precisely formed and polished. Because alumina is one of the hardest materials known, cutting requires diamond-tipped tools and polishing requires a diamond paste. Other ceramics which have been considered but not used for prostheses are similarly hard.

5 POROUS COMPONENTS

In metals, plastics or ceramics, porous components can be made by pressing a powder sufficiently to impose the shape of a component but not sufficiently to fill all the voids, and then heating the components sufficiently to cause the particles to adhere to each other but not sufficiently to fuse and obliterate the voids. The final porosity depends on close control of many factors such as the size and shape of the particles, the moulding pressure, and the temperature and time at temperature. Although the principles are common to the three types of material, the values of pressure and temperature needed will obviously be very different. With metals, an alternative technique is to take thin wire, and kink it and crush it to form a porous interlinked mass which can be given a permanent shape by being heated in the same way as used with metallic powder. This is the technique used by Galante et al. (1971). Another technique applicable to ceramics, and used by Klawitter and Hulbert (1971) and Lyng et al. (1973), is to mix the alumina or other powder in a liquid vehicle with other materials which, when heated, will react to form a gas and thereby make the mass porous. The paste can be cast into moulds and allowed to dry, leaving a component strong enough to be handled and heated.

All these techniques produce materials which are weak because the effective cross-sectional area is reduced, and brittle because a porous material is in effect composed of many stress concentrations joined together. Therefore the tendency is to apply porous coatings to metallic or plastic components, rather than to make the entire component porous. Ceramics are brittle even when not porous, and their tensile strength is sufficient to allow their use for only certain types of component. These factors make it desirable to use porous coatings rather than components which are porous all through.

REFERENCES

Galante, J., Rostoker, W., Lueck, R. and Ray, R. D. (1971) Sintered fiber metal composites as a basis for attachment of implants to bone. *Journal of Bone and Joint Surgery* **53A,** 101.

Klawitter, J. J. and Hulbert, S. F. (1971) Application of porous ceramics for the attachment of load bearing internal orthopaedic applications. *Journal of Biomedical Materials Research, Symposium No. 2*, part 1, pp. 161–229.

Lyng, S., Sudmann, E., Hulbert, S. F. and Sauer, B. W. (1973) Fixation of permanent orthopaedic prosthesis. Use of ceramics in the tibial-plateau. *Acta Orthopaedica Scandinavica* **44,** 694.

CHAPTER SEVEN

Standards, Control and Approval

1 PRELIMINARY CONSIDERATIONS

THE surgeon and the patient may ask for some assurance that joint replacement surgery will be successful; whether they ask for it or not, the information on which such an assurance could be based must be available. In order to examine what has to be done to produce any assurance about clinical success, the possible modes of failure must be considered.

In roughly the chronological order in which they might be expected to be apparent, these are:
death of patient;
infection;
limited function;
loosening;
corrosion;
fracture of the implant;
reaction to wear products;
wearing out.

Some of these, if of limited severity, need not constitute failure; but any one of them can leave the patient in such a state that the treatment must be regarded as having failed.

The factors on which these possible modes of failure depend are:
design;
materials;
manufacture;
surgery;
patient activity.

Two points are immediately apparent. Firstly, surgery and patient activity cannot be regulated in the same ways as can design, materials and manufacture. Secondly, none of the possible modes of failure is strictly uninfluenced by either surgery or patient activity. Resistance to corrosion depends mainly on the choice of material and manufacturing techniques, but can be reduced by surface damage sustained during implantation. The chance of death or infection occurring depends hardly at all on the implant itself and almost entirely on clinical factors. The remaining possible modes of failure all depend partly on the implant itself (design, material, manufacture) and partly on the use made of it (surgery, patient activity).

Thus any discussion of controls or standards must take account of the fact that for practical purposes all the possible modes of failure depend partly on factors which can be specified and verified in a reasonably precise way and partly on other factors which cannot. This being so, there is no possibility of guaranteeing 100 per cent clinical success. Whilst this is not a licence to make, for example, implants that will readily corrode, it does limit the precision which can meaningfully be embodied in some aspects of specifications.

Two other general considerations should be mentioned here. First, certain aspects of design, and all aspects of materials and manufacture, can be specified; but many of the tests which are used to verify that specified properties have been achieved are necessarily destructive and can therefore be performed on samples only. This means that assurances about the properties of implants other than those tested depend on assumptions about the consistency of all the processes involved. Second, only those features can be completely specified which are established and unlikely to be changed frequently; yet new designs, materials and manufacturing methods are certain to be introduced, and any system of specifications must ensure that products which purport to conform to established usage do so, while allowing innovations to be used sufficiently to show whether they ought or ought not to be accepted as standard practice.

The remainder of this chapter will consider, in the light of the above, what can be done to answer the questions which the surgeon or patient might ask.

2 QUESTIONS TO BE ANSWERED

A surgeon intending to use a design of prosthesis with which long clinical experience has been recorded must be assumed to have satisfied himself from the literature that the design is suitable for his purposes, that the clinical results achieved elsewhere are acceptable, etc. He therefore needs to know merely whether any particular example is in fact made to the design in question, and whether it has been made properly of the right materials. Each of these three matters can be controlled relatively easily.

A surgeon considering using a new design, i.e. one with which little or no clinical experience has been recorded, may want to know what preclinical efforts have been made to maximise the chance of clinical success. This amounts to asking for the results of laboratory tests of wear rate, strength of prosthetic components, strength of fixation, and joint function. If new materials are involved, the results of corrosion or compatibility tests are also relevant. All these tests can be performed, but the resulting information is not of the same kind as that concerning conformity to established practice.

Thus the surgeon should appreciate that the answers to his questions are in two groups: (1) those relating to established designs, materials and manufacturing methods, which can be expressed as assurances with known margins of error; and (2) those relating to new designs, materials or manufacturing methods, which consist of observations about which he must make his own judgement. The means of providing the answers can best be considered in relation to these two groups in turn.

3 ESTABLISHED DESIGNS, MATERIALS AND MANUFACTURING METHODS

3.1 General Requirements

It is necessary to have a specification and a means of verifying that products comply with the specification. This implies the existence of a body which compiles and issues specifications, and the existence of an organisation which can examine products and processes. 'Examination' may mean the scrutiny of manufacturing drawings, or the destructive or non-destructive testing of raw materials, semifinished products or finished products. The organisational implications are discussed later; this section deals with the practical aspects.

3.2 Designs

3.2.1 SPECIFICATIONS

Specifications in general can be grouped into those which specify the functions to be performed and those which specify some of the characteristics of the device which is to perform the functions. To take the analogy of the aeroplane, a specification of the first type would say that the aeroplane must carry a certain load at a certain speed and height, whilst one of the second type would say that the windows must be of a certain size and the upholstery of a certain colour, or the basic structure of a certain alloy. In dealing with established designs of joint prostheses, the matter is fairly simple: the size, shape and material are known, and can be specified as fully as desired by a combination of drawings and words. Thus the characteristics of the device are specified, and the functions need not be, on the assumption that if the characteristics are reproduced the functions, which have previously been observed, will also be reproduced.

3.2.2 VERIFICATION

Manufacturing drawings can be compared with master drawings for the design in question, and the product can be inspected to establish whether it complies with the manufacturing drawings. Dimensional inspection is non-destructive and can be performed on all products. In practice, it is common to inspect only certain critical dimensions on all products, and to inspect other dimensions on a sample basis.

3.3 Materials

3.3.1 SPECIFICATIONS

Established materials are easily dealt with. In all technologically advanced countries, nationally recognised bodies exist (British Standards Institution, American Society for Testing and Materials, etc.) which publish specifications for the composition, heat-treatment and mechanical properties of alloys. Specifications for special-purpose alloys are formulated and issued as necessary, and thus in all countries in which joint prostheses are manufactured, national specifications for the necessary alloys are available. The several national specifications for any one alloy are not usually identical, but are usually compatible, and some manufacturers operate their own internal specifications which are compatible with, but tighter than, the corresponding national specifications. Thus the difficulties resulting from the operations of several independent specifying authorities are less serious than might have been expected. Even so, there are moves towards a system of international specifications, issued by the International Standardisation Organisation, of which the national bodies mentioned above are members.

Plastics are less fully covered by specifications than are alloys. Since, as mentioned above, for many years virtually all plastic bearing surfaces in prostheses have been made of one grade of polyethylene produced by one manufacturer, that manufacturer's specification has perforce been accepted by all users.

Ceramics cannot yet be regarded as established prosthetic materials in the sense used here.

3.3.2 VERIFICATION

Whether a sample of alloy does or does not have the composition or mechanical properties specified is determined by straightforward tests. Since almost all these tests are necessarily destructive, they must obviously be done on a sample basis, and this immediately introduces two requirements: (1) that batches of material be identified and traceable throughout their manufacturing history; and (2) that the manufacturing processes be so consistent that the results of tests on samples can be relied on to represent the properties of the batch with a known margin of error. These requirements are accepted as normal in industries making precision products the performance of which can affect life or health, and such industries (e.g. the aircraft industry) have organisations and procedures designed for these purposes.

3.4 Manufacture

3.4.1 SPECIFICATIONS

Since manufacture of established designs is by nature a repetitive process, it can in principle be specified in every detail; such matters as the types of cutting tool and coolants, the exact heat-treatment sequences, or the type of polishing abrasive to be used can all be defined. Undesirable processes, such as the welding of stainless steel, can be prohibited, and processes thought to be necessary can be required.

It is also possible to specify the results obtained by the use of the specified processes, but the results depend on the design and material as well as on the processes. Thus any such specification, and any tests of conformity to it, must relate to all three. The mechanical properties or crystal structure of an alloy component in its finished state are obvious examples of characteristics in this category.

Verification of repetitive production processes is simple in principle, but to be fully effective demands either a large number of inspecting staff (and corresponding costs) or assurances that the processes are performed with enough consistency to make sample inspection acceptable.

4 NEW DESIGNS, MATERIALS AND MANUFACTURING METHODS

4.1 General Requirements

Some things which are new may be so in a technical sense only, and not in such a way as to affect the function of the implant; thus the first requirement is a means of deciding which innovations can be included under existing practice and which require testing. For those which require testing, the next requirement is to decide what tests should be performed and what results should be taken as justifying clinical use. This requirement applies to new designs, materials and manufacturing methods. An entirely new shape of prosthesis obviously requires testing; a new material or a new method of forming an existing material may be expected to give a reduced wear rate or higher strength, and these aspects of performance can be tested. Under this heading, the function of the implanted prosthesis (in the sense of the range(s) of movement conferred), its strength, the strength of its fixation to the bones, and the rate of wear of the bearing surfaces can all be tested in the laboratory.

4.2 Laboratory Testing

Static strength testing, of either prosthetic components by themselves or the prosthesis–bone system, requires straightforward equipment. For tests of prosthesis–bone systems, the well known uncertainties surrounding the use of dead and possibly unrepresentative bone add to the difficulties.

Fatigue testing of prosthetic components, if unidirectional load is applied, can be performed in standard and generally available equipment. This is still true if corrosion-fatigue tests, which are more useful, are required. If a more elaborate fatigue test, making some attempt to reproduce the ranges of loads and movements applied in life, is required, then clearly the situation is much more complicated.

A special-purpose machine is required; if, as is usual, it tests the two components of any one prosthesis in their intended mutual relationship, it is necessarily performing a wear test at the same time as a fatigue strength test. Such a device is called a simulator. To design and make a simulator is not in itself particularly difficult; as always in this field, the difficulty is in knowing whether all the test conditions imposed by the simulator are representative. Present knowledge of the loads arising in patients using joint prostheses and the relationships of these loads to movements is extremely limited. Worse, the loads actually arising in a prosthetic joint in life depend on the load-deformation characteristics of the body members through which the joint is loaded: in hip prostheses, for example, this means the stiffness, in every possible mode of loading, of everything from the ground to the pelvis. In a knee prosthesis, the factors contributing to the actual loads are nearly as many, and their effects probably greater because virtually all knee prostheses have in themselves some resistance to rotation about axes other than that of flexion–extension, and therefore forces can be generated which cannot arise in the usual spherical form of hip prosthesis. Clearly, wide variation between patients must be expected, and any one simulator test can simulate only one of a wide range of sets of loads and movements. The wear-testing aspect of a simulator test is attended by all these difficulties, in addition to those of wear testing in general (discussed in Chapter 3) compounded by the impossibility of using exactly the same fluid as is present in life.

A recent review by the present author (Swanson 1976) showed that, whilst at least 15 simulators exist in at least five countries (Table 7.1), few new or modified designs of prostheses appear to have been tested in simulators before being implanted in patients (Table 7.2); much of what has been learned from simulator tests either was already known or could have been learned from simpler tests, and no major feature of current practice has been derived from simulator tests. This apparently small return for the effort expended on simulators results largely from the difficulties, described above, of compiling a realistic specification for the performance of joint replacement prostheses.

Within the limitations discussed above, the results of laboratory testing can be used in certain ways, as follows.

The strength, particularly the fatigue strength, of the prosthetic components can be measured in the worst likely loading mode.

The static strength of the bone–prosthesis assembly can be measured.

The strengths measured in these two ways can be compared with the best available information, which may be:

the loads applied in life (where these are known);

the corresponding strengths measured on natural joints; or

the corresponding strengths measured on established prostheses.

The mode of failure when overloaded can be observed, particularly whether it involves fracture of a prosthetic component, loosening, fracture of a bone, or a reversible subluxation.

The rate of wear can be measured and compared with that measured in other prostheses, preferably established designs.

4.3 Making Specifications

The purpose of laboratory testing is to provide information which will help a surgeon to decide whether, and in what circumstances, to use a particular prosthesis. For this purpose, some of the tests suggested above produce results which are self-explanatory (e.g. the range of movement or the mode of failure in overload) but others produce results which must be evaluated to be useful. Ultimately somebody must decide that a given result is or is not acceptable as a basis for clinical use, and this amounts to preparing a specification, even if an informal one. At the time of writing, a new hip prosthesis (whether new in geometry, material or manufacture) could be compared, in respect of strength, wear rate and mode of failure, with established hip prostheses tested in the same conditions; but this

Table 7.1 Simulators Mentioned in Publications

Location of simulator	First mentioned
Stanmore, England	Mk 1: Scales, Duff-Barclay and Burrows 1965
	Mk 2: Scales and Wright 1975
Leeds, England	Walker et al. 1969
Hospital for Special Surgery, New York, USA	Walker and Gold 1971
Cincinatti, Ohio, USA	Dumbleton, Miller and Miller 1972
Imperial College, London, England	Freeman, Swanson and Heath 1972
Lyon, France	Bousquet and Grammont 1972
MIT, Cambridge, Mass., USA	Weightman et al. 1972
Pau, France	Boutin 1972
Winterthur, Switzerland (Sulzer Brothers)	Weber and Semlitsch 1972
Cachan, France (Benoist Girard)	Lagrange and Letournel 1973
Grand Rapids, Mich., USA	Swanson 1973
GUEPAR, France	Aubriot, Deburge and Schramm 1973
Irvine, Calif., USA	Waugh et al. 1973
München, Germany	Ungethüm et al. 1973
Syracuse, New York, USA	Shaw and Murray 1973

Table 7.2 Simulator Tests Mentioned in Connection with Particular Designs

Symposium	Designs used in patients	Designs by owners of simulators	Designs tested in simulators
Total Hip Replacement, Clinical Orthopaedics, Sept.–Oct., 1970	8	1	0
Arthroplasty of the Hip, edited by Chapchal, 1972	3	2	2
Arthroplastie du Genou, Acta Orthopaedica Belgica, Jan.–Feb., 1973	11	6	3
Total Knee Replacement, Clinical Orthopaedics, July–Aug., 1973	12	4	3
Total Knee Replacement, Institution of Mechanical Engineers, Sept., 1974	15	4	1

would not be possible with a prosthesis for any other joint. For any other joint, the best that could be done would be to compare the results with, for example, the strength of the natural joint or the wear rate of an established hip prosthesis. The discussions of stresses in prosthetic components and the influence of fixation (Chapter 2, section 3.2) and of wear testing (Chapter 3) showed that many experimental factors must be controlled if the results of different tests are to be validly compared.

It may therefore be concluded that at the present time, for all joints other than the hip, it is unrealistic to prepare specifications more detailed than necessary to exclude the obviously unsafe, and that laboratory testing is limited to producing results which will show that a prosthesis is apparently reasonably safe. On this basis, a surgeon or body of surgeons must decide whether or not to proceed to clinical trials. For the hip, the existence of established designs means that their strengths and wear rates could be made the limits for acceptance of new or modified designs when tested in the same conditions. As experience is accumulated at other joints, this possibility may extend to them. As in other fields of engineering, when the phenomena concerned are sufficiently understood it may be possible to dispense with some measurements of performance because the performance can be reliably predicted from characteristics which can be more easily verified. For example, when the wear process is more fully understood it may be possible to say that a certain surface finish and accuracy of fit will lead to a known rate of wear in a given material when subjected to a given range of stress. It would then be possible simply to require those characteristics to be within specified ranges, and some wear tests could then be dispensed with. For most aspects of performance, however, some testing of the final product, which encompasses the design, the materials and the manufacturing methods, will always be wanted as an assurance.

5 ORGANISATION AND ENFORCEMENT

It seems to be widely accepted that, in a branch of surgery which relies as heavily as this one does on devices with a high technological content, some control is necessary.

From the above, it appears that, if any control at all is to be exercised, in any country in which prostheses are manufactured and used some organisation is needed which will publish specifications covering design, materials and manufacture and make some attempt to ensure that the specifications are followed. In a country in which prostheses are used but not manufactured, the control can be exercised only indirectly, by deciding which of other countries' products to admit.

The evaluation of test results for new designs, materials and manufacturing methods could in principle be done by each interested clinician for himself, but most such people would welcome at least some guidance from a body having available the necessary surgical and engineering expertise. This suggests that in each country concerned a national body is needed for this purpose. It seems desirable to incorporate in new developments the lessons from clinical experience as it is accumulated, and this suggests a process of continuous review, with particular attention to failures. It is important to know whether failures, either sudden or gradual, are attributable to design, to characteristics of the material or manufacture of a particular batch of implants, or to mis-use. This means that information about failures is of limited use unless it includes a knowledge of the complete manufacturing and clinical history of the implant concerned. This in turn means that every implant should carry a serial number which can be related, through manufacturers' records, to material and manufacturing batches, and that full clinical records must be available for every case. It is obvious that a central body attempting to use the results of experience to guide future design cannot be fully effective unless it receives the fullest possible feedback of information about clinical experience, particularly failures. This introduces the notion of some sort of compulsion on clinicians to report failures in detail and results in general. The implementation of such a policy would be intrusive, expensive and laborious, and one must ask whether the benefits would match the cost. In this connection it should be noted that a high proportion of failures (in the broad sense of the term, as defined at the beginning of this chapter) are due to clinical or surgical factors, and that where failure is attributable at least partly to the prosthesis, such as the excessive rate of wear of PTFE acetabular cups or the fatigue fracture of femoral component stems in prosthetic hips, the remedial action, while it may or may not be easy to take, is easily identified without the need for vast numbers of specimens to be examined in detail.

Whatever body attempts to approve designs must have the confidence of the orthopaedic profession in the country concerned. In most countries, the involvement of central government in the provision of health care is such that the approving body must also be acceptable to the relevant government department and perhaps formally part of it.

The approval and inspection of materials and manufacture is less a matter for the orthopaedic profession and more one for the engineering profession and the industry. From what has been said above, it is clear that inspection or testing of samples by representatives of any organisation is inadequate unless the whole manufacturing process, from the making of the alloy to the packing of the finished prostheses, is organised and controlled so as to guarantee that any particular characteristic of the product will vary from a sample value within known limits. This is the requirement underlying the concept of 'quality assurance', and it can be achieved only within the industry; external inspectors can detect bad products, but they cannot make a bad industry able to manufacture good products. This having been said, in the aircraft industry (which has already been used as a basis for comparison) the need for monitoring of quality by an organisation separate from the manufacturer is universally accepted, and in all countries in which prostheses are manufactured or likely to be there are organisations possessing the necessary experience and recognised by governments, customers (where these are separate from governments) and the industry concerned. Since the requirements for the control of quality of prostheses are so similar to those for aircraft components, it seems sensible to try to use the expertise of these existing organisations.

In many countries, legislation allows the relevant central government department to control by regulation any substance or device used in the treatment of patients, and therefore in those countries all the matters which have been discussed in this chapter could become matters of law. In practice, the staff of those government departments in most countries concerned have refrained from making regulations as widely as they might, and have encouraged the orthopaedic and engineering professions to co-operate in preparing such schemes for approval and control as have been advanced. Bearing in mind that the final act in the sequence, the decision by the surgeon about what to implant and how, is most unlikely ever to be controlled by legislation more detailed than that requiring proper professional competence and care, it would be out of proportion to apply the full apparatus of the law to the earlier acts, which can be sufficiently controlled by agreement between all the parties.

In any field of activity where safety is important and resources are finite, there is a problem in deciding what effort to spend on control. Everybody would agree that obviously unsuitable materials or dangerous implants should not be available to the surgeon. At the other end of the scale, the message of this chapter is that in this field 100 per cent success can never be guaranteed. If 100 per cent success is unattainable, governments and the professions concerned must be careful that they do not, for reasons of bureaucratic seemliness, allow themselves to become involved in time-consuming and intrusive procedures which produce little measurable benefit in terms of over-all safety for the patient.

REFERENCES

Aubriot, J. H., Deburge, A. and Schramm, P. (1973) La prothèse Guepar. *Acta Orthopaedica Belgica* **39,** 257.

Bousquet, G. and Grammont, P. (1972) Etude expérimentale de la longevité des prothèses de hanche du point de vue mécanique. *Acta Orthopaedica Belgica* **38,** Suppl. 1, 123.

Boutin, P. (1972) Arthroplastie total de la hanche par prothèse en alumine frittée. *Revue de Chirurgie Orthopédique et Reparatrice de l'Appareil Moteur* **58,** 229.

Chapchal, G. (ed.) (1972) *Arthroplasty of the Hip*. Stuttgart, Thieme.

Dumbleton, J. H., Miller, D. A. and Miller, E. H. (1972) A simulator for load bearing joints. *Wear* **20,** 165.

Freeman, M. A. R., Swanson, S. A. V. and Heath, J. C. (1972) Biological properties of the wear particles generated by all cobalt–chrome total joint replacement prostheses. In, *Arthroplasty of the Hip*, p. 8. Ed. G. Chapchal. Stuttgart, Thieme.

Lagrange, J. and Letournel, E. (1973) Principes et réalisation de la prothèse totale de genou 'LL'. *Acta Orthopaedica Belgica* **39,** 280.

Scales, J. T. and Wright, K. W. J. (1975) Experimental methods for the assessment of wear of materials potentially useful for endoprostheses. *Acta Orthopaedica Belgica* **41,** Suppl. 1, 160.

Scales, J. T., Duff-Barclay, I. and Burrows, H. J. (1965) Some engineering and medical problems associated with massive bone replacement. In, *Biomechanics and Related Bio-Engineering Topics*, p. 205. Ed. R. M. Kenedi. Oxford, Pergamon.

Shaw, J. A. and Murray, D. G. (1973) Knee joint simulator. *Clinical Orthopaedics and Related Research* **94,** 15.

Swanson, A. B. (1973) Low modulus force-dampening materials for knee joint prostheses. *Acta Orthopaedica Belgica* **39,** 116.

Swanson, S. A. V. (1976) The limitations of simulators. In, 'The Evaluation of Artificial Joints with particular reference to Joint Simulators', Conference held in Leeds, 16 January 1976. Ed. V. Wright. (to be published)

Ungethüm, M., Hildebrandt, J., Jäger, M. and Moslé, H. G. (1973) Ein neuer Simulator zur Testung von Totalendoprothesen für das Hüftgelenk. *Archiv für Orthopädische und Unfall-Chirurgie* **77,** 304.

Walker, P. S. and Gold, B. L. (1971) The tribology (friction, lubrication and wear) of all-metal artificial hip joints. *Wear* **17,** 285.

Walker, P. S., Dowson, D., Longfield, M. D. and Wright, V. (1969) A joint simulator. In, *Lubrication and Wear in Joints*, p. 104. Ed. V. Wright. London, Sector Publ.

Waugh, T. R., Smith, R. C., Orofino, C. F. and Anzel, S. M. (1973) Total knee replacement. Operative technic and preliminary results. *Clinical*

Orthopaedics and Related Research **94**, 196.

Weber, B. G. and Semlitsch, M. (1972) Total hip replacement with rotation-endoprosthesis. Problem of wear. In, *Arthroplasty of the Hip*, p. 71. Ed. G. Chapchal. Stuttgart, Thieme.

Weightman, B. O., Simon, S., Paul, I. L., Rose, R. and Radin, E. L. (1972) Lubrication mechanism of hip joint replacement prostheses. *Journal of Lubrication Technology (ASME)* **94**, 131.

Index

compressive strength, 3, 9
  of joint replacement materials, 11,12
corrosion
  crevice, 7
  electrochemical nature of, 8
  galvanic, 7
  of joint replacement materials, 13–14
  surface blemishes as foci of, 162
corrosion-fatigue, 5, 8
  of joint replacement materials, 14–15
crack propagation, 3, 6
creep, 3, 10
cyclohexyl methacrylate, 153
cysts, 98, 135

DEGRADATION
  of ceramics and polymers, 8
  of joint replacement materials, 14, 16, 69, 70, 72
degradative fatigue, 8
  of joint replacement materials, 15
Delrin, *see* polyacetal
ductility, 2, 3

ELASTIC limit, 2
elastic modulus, *see* Young's modulus *and* shear modulus
elbow prostheses, *see* prostheses

FAILURE, causes of, after joint replacement, 167
failures, information about, 174–5
fatigue
  fracture, 6
    of femoral stems, 12–13, 36–7
  limit, 5
  of dead bone, 96, 112
  strength, 5
    of joint replacement materials 11, 12
    of prosthesis–bone interface, 131
  test, 4–5
fenestration of stem, 97, 145
finite element analysis, 34
fixation
  acceptable, definition of, 131
  by bone ingrowth, 97–101, 144–7
  by cement, *see* cement
  by interference fit, 139
  by interlock, 142–4
  by nuts and bolts, 141
  by screws, 44, 139–40, 143
  mechanics of, 130–55
  of individual prostheses, *see* prostheses
flange, 137, 138
Fluon, *see* polytetrafluorethylene

forging
  of steel and titanium alloys, 160
  reason for using, 159
fracture, 2, 3
  brittle, 3
  ductile, 3
  fatigue, 6
    of femoral stems, 12–13, 36–8
  stress, at, 2, 34
friction
  fundamentals of
    coefficient of, 47
    effect of lubrication on, 53, 54
    effect of sliding speed on, 47, 48, 54
    effect of surface finish on, 48, 54
    laws of, 47
    'stiction', 48
  of total joint replacement materials
    effect of geometry on, 62, 65, 66, 67
    effect of lubrication on, 63
    effect of size on, 65, 66, 67, 72
    effect of surface finish on, 62, 66–67
    in joint simulators, 61–8
    in simple machines, 55–61
    'stiction', 65

GLASS-CERAMIC implants, 147
grinding, 161

HAIR, chromium in, 102
hardness
  in friction and wear, 4, 47–9 (*see also* wear equations)
  of joint replacement materials, 11
  tests, 4
heat treatment of cast components, 161
hinged prostheses, 134
  stresses on stems, 43
hip prostheses, *see* prostheses

IMPLANT materials, 9–16
  mechanical properties of, 11–12, 151–2
  see also particular materials
infection
  prosthetic design and, 122
  wear debris and, 123
ingrowth of bone, *see* bone
inspection
  dimensional, 169
  limitations of, 175
interface, bone–implant, *see* bone; fixation; loosening; *and* soft tissue
interference fit, 139

interlock
  by bone ingrowth, 145–7
  by gross shape of implant, 142–4
  complementary to use of cement, 144
  to transmit shear or torsion, 143–4
  to transmit tension or compression, 142–3
International Standardisation Organisation, 170
intramedullary stems
  cross-sectional shape, 138
  see also stem *and* stress analysis
investment casting, 160–1
iron in tissues, 106

KNEE prostheses, *see* prostheses

LABORATORY testing, 171–2
load
  on normal joints, 133
  transfer of at bone–implant interface, 130–55
loosening
  bone death and, 112–17
  mechanics of, 130–55
  tissue response and, 114–22
  wear debris and, 114–22
lost wax casting process, 160–1
lubrication
  fundamentals of
    boundary, 53, 54
    elastohydrodynamic, 53
    fluid, 53, 54
    hydrodynamic, 53
    squeeze-film, 53
  of total joint replacement materials
    in joint simulators, 61–8
    in simple machines, 55–61

MARKING of components, 162
metal-to-metal prostheses, and skin sensitivity, 118–21
metal sensitivity, 117–22
methyl methacrylate, *see* cement
modulus of elasticity, *see* Young's modulus *and* shear modulus
molybdenum particles, 115
moulding of plastic components, 164, 165
MP 35 N, *see* cobalt–nickel alloy

NEOPLASIA, 124–5
neutral axis, 20, 21, 22
nickel
  constituent of alloys, 9, 112
  in tissues, 111, 112, 121
  particles, 115
  sensitivity to, 117, 118
Nylon, *see* polyamide